HEALTHY KNEES CYCLING

ROBIN ROBERTSON

HEALTHY KNEES CYCLING

The Fun No-Impact Way to Reduce Joint Pain, Improve Strength, and Help You Live an Active Lifestyle.

USA Cycling Coach Level 2, Functional Aging Specialist, ACE Certified Personal Training, Owner and Manager Bellingham Tennis Club and Fairhaven Fitness, Creator of Cycle Moles and Healthy Knees Coach.

Publishing support, design, and composition by Nicole Gebhardt and team: Marketing and communications solutions for niche experts. www.BookItAuthors.com

Disclaimer:
Not all exercises are suitable for everyone and this or any other exercise program may result in injury. To reduce risk of injury, consult your physician before beginning this exercise program. The creators, producers, participants and distributors of this program disclaim any liabilities or loss in connection with the exercise, the equipment used, and/or herein.

ISBN-10: 0-692-59770-0
ISBN-13: 978-0-692-59770-5

DEDICATION

For my high school running coach, Mr. Brock Hogle, who inspired me to dig deep and do more than I thought I could. He taught me mental toughness and always inspired my individual capabilities and our team.

For my many skilled medical practitioners…thank you for the superb care you have given to me through my life time of knee issues to keep my body working well. I am thankful!

A special thanks for my parents, Frank and Elena Mortimer, who had a knack of showing love and support throughout my life. They allowed me to get a paper route in 6th grade so that I could save money to buy my first 10-speed bike and also gave me my life-saving road bike in college after I got the news that I could no longer run.

And of course, for my handsome husband and best friend, Doug Robertson, an extraordinary man who always believes in me. Your support for my wild ideas means the world to me. I wouldn't trade any of our adventures for anything and look forward to many more years of fun on (and off!) our bikes together. And for my children, Elena and Foster, for putting up with my cycling stories and knee complaints all these years, and for the love you have given to me. I couldn't do any of this without the three of you.

TABLE OF CONTENTS

PREFACE

By Robin Robertson

My knee problems? I was born with them. All of my knee troubles stemmed from being born with abnormally shaped meniscus cartilage in both knees. I've had eight knee surgeries (to date) and still have my own knees. I know about knee pain because I've had it all my life.

Yet I've managed to stay fit and active because I've learned how to take care of my knees along the way. It took me 25 years to learn the secrets in this book. I want to give you a shortcut to relieving your knee pain and feeling better. Why do I want to share this with you? Because I know it's no fun to live with pain. I want to give you hope there is a way to regain an active and healthy life.

Now, my knee story. My knees always hurt, even when I was little. When I straightened my left leg, it would "ka-lunk" and shift and sometimes my knee would lock or sometimes it would give out. I fell down a lot as a kid. It confounded doctors for years as to what was wrong because an x-ray only shows bone (and MRI technology hadn't been invented). Finally, I had a procedure called an "arthrogram" where dye was injected in my knee to stain the cartilage so it would be visible on an x-ray.

I was diagnosed with a discoid meniscus: instead of a "C" shape, the meniscus was shaped like a filled in "D" with a lump in it. I received the standard open knee surgery to remove <u>ALL</u> of the meniscus cartilage on the outside of my left knee because that was the technology at the time. My doctor told me to exercise as tolerated by pain. I was just 13 years old.

I learned to tolerate a lot of pain so I could be active. I was an avid downhill skier and ran competitively in high school and college. What I didn't know: I was actually damaging my knee through these activities.

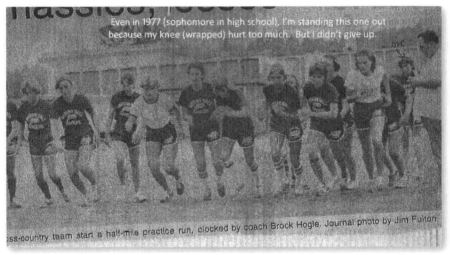

Even in 1977 (sophomore in high school), I'm standing this one out because my knee (wrapped) hurt too much. But I didn't give up.

oss-country team start a half-mile practice run, clocked by coach Brock Hogle. Journal photo by Jim Fulton.

Robin High School Track

My second knee surgery was in the winter of my senior year in college. I had finished the cross-country running season and was about to enter my final track season but my knee was so painful I had to do something. After the surgery, my doctor told me if he didn't know how old I was, he'd think I was about 85 for the amount of arthritis in my knee. He told me, "If you want to walk at age 30, you must stop ALL impact sports right away." He showed me the video of the surgery and I could plainly see one side of my knee had healthy cartilage and bones and the other side looked like someone had taken a jackhammer to the surface. BOOM! My world shifted. At age 24, I learned I had severe osteoarthritis.

After that, it wasn't such a hard decision to quit running. I had already stopped skiing because it hurt more than it was fun. I now knew running wasn't just about being tough enough to put up with the pain. I was doing real and irreversible damage to my knee. But I certainly couldn't stop everything and do nothing. "NO" is not a solution to me, so I switched to bicycling and found an entirely new joy in life.

The prediction eventually came true: at age 34 years old, I could hardly walk around the block, even though I had stopped impact activities. Basic daily activities were painful and even cycling was getting uncomfortable. I went Christmas shopping on crutches with a backpack so I didn't use my knee. The scariest part was I could not chase after my kids who were two and four years old. I couldn't even walk them to the swings in the park just 2 ½ blocks away. This made me cry! I cried for the pain and I cried for my loss of ability.

My knee was deforming (angulating), making me quite knock-kneed in my left leg. The more knock-kneed I became, the more my body weight was driving through the damaged part of the joint, and the faster the damage (and pain) mounted. I limped badly. Every step was excruciating.

I was told I needed a knee replacement but I was too young (for how long the joints were lasting and how many times they could be replaced). Luckily, there was an alternative. I underwent a "femoral osteotomy" where my thigh bone was cut and re-aligned. I was no longer knock-kneed. It was a long recovery with three months no-weight bearing on crutches. About a year post surgery, I remember taking a step and, for the first time I could remember, feeling no pain. Ah, a miracle!

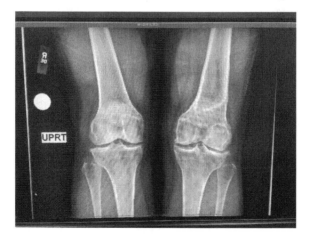

Robin's knee X-ray 2015

I've had three additional surgeries on that same knee, primarily to remove arthritic bone spurs that were inhibiting joint movement plus some cartilage clean up on the other side of my knee.

My "good knee" was not without its own problems. The two surgeries on my right knee were to arthroscopically (three small incisions in the knee instead of the open knee surgery) trim out the deformed cartilage and remove some fragments that were causing my knee to lock up. I don't dwell on the fact that if arthroscopic surgery had been possible for my left knee, my life would be different. My right knee has always been my workhorse, compensating for the left. At current, it is also arthritic, but not quite as advanced as the other.

In addition to all of the surgeries, I've had injections with cortisone, hyaluronic acid (viscosupplementation), and platelet rich plasma (PRP) to varying degrees of pain relief.

I know I am still active, healthy, and happy because I turned to cycling. This non-impact sport builds the muscles in my legs, keeps my heart strong, and gives me stress relief. About a year ago, my orthopedic surgeon told me if it weren't for cycling and staying light weight (yes, I must work at that too), I would have had to replace my knee ten years ago. This statement resonated with me and gave me the inspiration to share what I know about reducing knee pain to live a healthy, active life.

INTRODUCTION

By Dr. Michael A Thorpe, MD

Michael A Thorpe, MD, is an orthopaedic surgeon with over 30 years medical experience. He specializes in out-patient surgery and sports medicine, having been the Team Orthopaedic Surgeon for Western Washington University since he arrived in Bellingham, Washington in 1988. Because he was a three-sport Division I college athlete, he understands the unique issues of the injured athlete. Knee, shoulder and hip problems dominate his practice, but he also performs routine foot and hand surgery, and emphasizes non-operative care of all problems, if applicable. Dr. Thorpe understands joint pain and rehabilitation, having been a competitive athlete, now with both of his own hips replaced. He received the Patient's Choice Award in 2011 and Washington State's Best Doctors Award in 2010 and 2013.

As an orthopedic surgeon, I think about solving joint problems every minute of my working day. My office shelves contain models of hip, knee, and shoulder replacement implants. In her new book, *Healthy Knees Cycling*, Robin Robertson brings a refreshing perspective on how a bicycle can help solve knee problems without surgery (hip and ankle problems, too).

Since starting my orthopedic practice in 1988, I have performed numerous knee surgeries including thousands of joint replacements. In 2006, I developed the first outpatient surgery center joint replacement program in the State of Washington. It is an alternative to hospitalization for the younger, healthier patients requiring hip, knee, or shoulder replacements and utilizes a one-night stay combined with home therapy.

Is knee surgery unavoidable? You and your doctor will make this decision together, depending on your pain and level of knee dysfunction.

It is sometimes possible to reduce pain to an acceptable level without surgery by strengthening the knee and surrounding structures. This avoids high costs, potential complications, and the necessary down time. Robin presents a sound method to do this with *Healthy Knees Cycling*. Even if knee replacement or other surgery is inevitable, the time and effort put towards strengthening your knee and leg muscles prior to surgery will greatly benefit you afterwards by quickening your recovery.

Robin Robertson has been my patient for many years. She first presented me, in 1995, a bone-on-bone arthritic knee. If she had been older, I would have recommended knee replacement. Robin was only 34-years-old at the time. Her knee was bringing her activity to a standstill. The pain was so great, Robin and I elected to proceed with a surgery to re-align her leg. When standing, her body weight no longer passed through the damaged side of her knee joint, but through the healthy side. I told her the benefits from this surgery may last 7 to 10 years before knee replacement might be necessary. I also advised non-weight-bearing exercise instead of running or walking. Now, twenty years later, Robin still has her own knee. I told her recently that if it weren't for bicycling and staying fit and light, we would have replaced her knee 10 years ago.

Bicycling is one of the best ways to strengthen your knee joint and the supporting muscles, tendons, and ligaments. With cycling, there is no lateral movement, only minimal weight bearing, and you receive the benefits of knee motion. Putting joints through a range of motion without impact nourishes the articular cartilage and improves its health. Your muscles, tendons, ligaments, and bones get stronger from this activity, which diminishes your pain.

But not everyone knows how to set up a bike, use good body form, and be smart about how fast to pedal and how much tension you should have in each pedal stroke. Robin's book is a gold mine of information for anyone wanting to improve knee health, reduce pain, lose weight, and hopefully avoid or delay surgery. Read it cover-to-cover and to get one for your fitness trainer as well if he/she isn't a certified Healthy Knees coach.

CHAPTER ONE

Knee Pain: What Does It Mean?

L et's cut to the chase. You picked up this book because your knees hurt or you know someone else whose knees hurt. I know a lot about knee pain. I was born with my knee problems and my knees have hurt as far back as I can remember. Knee pain has always been a part of my life to lesser and greater degrees. Unknowingly, I did activities that caused irreversible damage. I have since learned I can choose (and so can you) to make better choices for knees to keep them healthier and reduce pain.

I want to help you along this Healthy Knee path as well. Knee pain is one of the most common grumbles. About one third of all doctor visits for muscle or bone pain are complaints about the knees[1].

In this first stage, we explore some anatomy so you know basic terms and the elements making up the knee. Next, we look at range of motion and what it takes to ride a bike. Last, I explain some of the causes of knee pain because you commonly hear these terms and I want you to know what they mean. This information should *not* be used as a diagnostic tool and I encourage you to seek medical help if your discomfort is persistent.

Knee Anatomy[2] – What is in your Knee?

Your knee is a weight-bearing joint that acts like a complex hinge. Your bones are your lever arms, your knee joint is the fulcrum (the center of rotation), and your muscles are the pulleys.

---

[1] WebMD (2015) *What's Causing your Knee Pain.* Retrieved on 11/11/15 from **http://www.webmd.com/pain-management/knee-pain/knee-pain-causes**

[2] For a more scientific and detailed description of the knee, please see the appendix.

Your bones are the support beams giving your body structure (without bones, you'd be a blob on the floor). Your knee joint is made up of three major bones: thigh bone (femur), shin bone (tibia), and knee cap (patella). Your lower leg also has a second smaller bone (fibula). It is beside the tibia and ends at the outside ankle.

Cartilage protects your bones. There are two types: the ends of bones are covered by a shrink-wrap padding of articular cartilage; between the femur and tibia bones are the shock absorbing and stabilizing cartilage cushions called the menisci (plural for meniscus). Positions on your body are referred to as "medial" or toward your midline and "lateral" as away from the midline (or to your side). You have a medial ("in" side of knee) and lateral ("out" side of knee) meniscus.

Synovial fluid is your joint oil. This olive oil-like viscous substance lubricates your joint and nourishes your cartilage. Synovial fluid just doesn't wander around in your knee; it is contained by the lining of the joint capsule.

Ligaments are the "ropes" tying your bones together. They stabilize your knee and keep it in the correct shape and position.

Tendons are the "ropes" fastening muscles to bone.

Knee Range of Motion and What You Need to Pedal

Your knee needs the ability to bend and straighten a certain amount when you ride a bike. How far does your knee straighten and bend? The normal range of motion for a knee is 0 degrees (straight) to fully flexed at 130-140 degrees (calf touching hamstring)[3]. Limited range of motion refers to a joint which, for some reason, has less than this full range of motion. This limited range of motion may cause you pain if you continually stress the upper and lower limits.

---

3   Normal Ranges of Joint Motion, Retrieved 8/24/15 from **http://web.mit.edu/tkd/stretch/stretching_8. html**

Range of Motion Needed to Ride a Bike = 25 degrees – 110 degrees

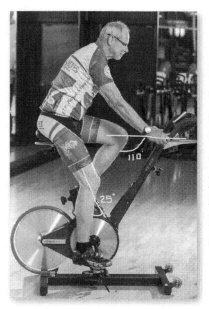

Here's the most important bit for riding a bike: you need a range of about 25 degrees (leg extended) to 110 degrees (leg bent) to make a full pedal rotation on your bike and be in the proper position. If you are recovering from an injury or surgery and you do not yet have this range, please see your doctor or physical therapist!

25 degrees looks like this: If you are sitting on the floor with your legs extended in front of you, a 25 degree bend is just about enough space to put your fist underneath your knee. Here is what it looks like on a bike:

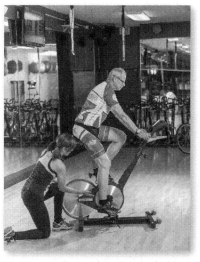

25 to 35 degree bend extended leg

A 110 degree bend is just past a right angle with your heel being closer to your hamstring than at 90 degrees.

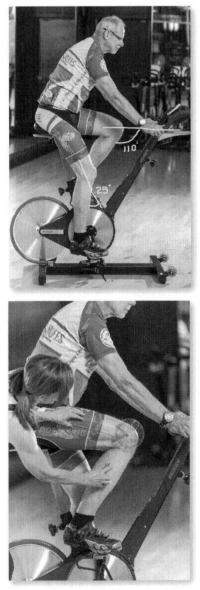

110 degree bend in knee at top of pedal stroke

Caution: if you are hoping to ride your bike (inside or out) and do not yet have the needed range of motion for your knee, you might be tempted to raise the saddle height so you can complete a full pedal stroke and bend your knee a little less. However, that may compromise your hips or lower back because your saddle height is too high and forces you to extend your knee (become more straight) at the bottom of the pedal stroke (so you can reach your pedal). When your saddle is too high, you may need to rock your hips on each pedal stroke for your foot to reach the pedal. This puts significant stress on your lower back.

That said, I have recovered from many surgeries with the aid of my bike. You can use the bike to regain the range of motion you need for pedaling. I have found it to be a combination of hard work, sometimes painful, and yet soothing. It feels good to work on the range of motion, somewhat like oiling a rusty hinge. Just be careful and use the guidance of your doctor or physical therapist (and don't fudge the saddle height.)

Common Causes of Knee Pain
Youze hurting me!

In his nightly bath at age two, my son would say "Youze hurting me!" if he got soap in his eyes. Plain and simple…there is pain, please make it stop.

Physical pain is your body's way of warning you about an injury. Your peripheral nerves send a signal from the affected area to your brain transmitting the information. Depending on the situation, this information may trigger an immediate response ("Get away!" or "Fight!") or may be part of the ongoing healing process. It could also be a whole host of responses somewhere in between.

As a part of healing, your body undergoes an immune response to an injury causing inflammation. Inflammation is like the aid car coming to the rescue and responds specifically to the type of injury you've received (think cut, bee sting, broken bone, overuse injury like tennis elbow). After the area is healed, inflammation goes away and the nervous system returns to normal. If the area cannot heal (as with arthritis), inflammation sticks around to continue its effort to heal.

Signs of inflammation and their causes include (2013)[4]
- Redness (increase in blood flow)
- Heat (increase in blood flow and metabolic activity)
- Swelling (increase in fluid loss from capillaries into the space between cells)
- Pain (stimulation of your neural pain receptors from compression due to swelling, chemical reactions, or infection.)
- Loss of Function (severe cases of inflammation due to swelling and pain.)

---

[4] McKinley, M, Dean O'Loughlin, V, Stouter Bidel, T. (2013) Anatomy and Physiology: An Integrative Approach, McGraw-Hill Companies.

Are you Sore or Injured?

Soreness is a natural part of muscle recovery from stressing the tissue beyond its normal activity. *Injury* is far more serious and may require treatment from a medical professional. Knowing the difference between the two is vital to maintaining an active and healthy life.

As you exercise, your muscles are put under strain. If this strain is greater than their usual load, the activity may cause micro tears in the muscle leaving inflammation and soreness to follow. This is good! This is normal! This is how you get stronger as your muscle rebuilds. After a few days the soreness should decrease dramatically.

If the soreness persists for longer or if you have sharp pain or restriction in movement, you may have crossed the line to injury. If you've had some sort of traumatic event (a fall, an automobile accident), or if you are suspicious of injury, you should always see your medical professional.

Why Pay Attention to Pain?

Pain is your caution light. It is telling you are in jeopardy of being injured.

I recommend you replace the saying "No pain, no gain" with "If it hurts, don't do it."

If you feel pain during a movement, you may be performing the exercise incorrectly, using too much weight, or the exercise is just not meant for you. Pain may also indicate you are aggravating an existing injury.

"If it hurts, don't do it" is different from "This is hard." The way you get stronger is through progressive overload or doing different activities. With progressive overload, you stress your muscles a little bit each time you exercise; you continue to get stronger. In cycling, you may work a little harder, ride a little longer, or use a different gear to change how your muscles are working.

Two Types of Knee Pain: On Bike Only, Off Bike All of the Time

Let's distinguish between two types of knee pain: pain you ONLY feel when you are on a bike (otherwise your knees feel pretty good) and knee pain you feel all the time.

Knee Pain on Bike Only

What if you only experience knee pain when you are ON your bike?

More than likely your knee pain is caused by your bike set up or the wrong sized frame on your bike. If you want to be comfortable on your bike, I highly recommend you invest in a professional bike fit. It is amazing how much a quarter of an inch fine-tuning can change your entire experience on a bike. For minor adjustments, read the Chapter 6 "Healthy Knees Secrets to Cycling" section to learn how to correct your bike set up for these issues.

Top of Knee Pain

If you feel pain at the top of your knee, your saddle height may be too low. This pain is primarily felt when you are pushing down on the pedals.

To explain why this happens requires a small anatomy lesson. Your four quadriceps muscles are all connected by a common tendon which includes your kneecap imbedded within it. Technically speaking, the tendon above the kneecap is called the quadriceps tendon and below the kneecap is the patellar tendon connecting the whole quadriceps group to the tibia in your lower leg.

When your saddle is too low, your thigh bone (femur) pushes forward over the bottom half of your knee (tibial plateau) putting stress on your quads and the attaching tendons (1991)[5].

---

[5]   Wozniak Timmer, C. (1991) Cycling Biomechanics: A Literature Review. JOSPT vol 14, No 3. Retrieved 8/24/15 from **http://www.jospt.org/doi/pdfplus/10.2519/jospt.1991.14.3.106**

The Suspect: Saddle Too Low

The Fix: Raise your saddle height so you have a 25-35 degree bend in your knee when your leg is at full extension.

Front of Knee Pain (kneecap area)

If you feel pain at the front of your knee, your saddle may be too close to your handlebars forcing your knee past your toes when your pedals are parallel to the ground.

Again, like in the description above, the pain is likely due to the pressure of your thigh bone pressing toward your knee cap as your knee is in the most forward part of the pedal stroke.

The Suspect: Saddle Too Close to Handlebars

The Fix: Move your saddle away from your handlebars. When you are sitting on your saddle with your feet parallel to the ground, the knee of your forward leg should not go past the point at which the pedal connects to the pedal arm. When you look down, you should be able to see the front 1/3 of your foot (ball of foot to your toes). If you were to hang a plumb-bob from your knee, the weight should hover over the center of the pedal and the ball of your foot.

If you adjust your saddle and now can see MORE than the front 1/3 of your foot, you've scooted it too far back.

Back of Pain Knee (and possibly your lower back)

Back of knee pain often indicates your seat is too high and you may be hyperextending your knee. The pain comes from overextending your leg.

Remember, you'll want to maintain a nice, slight bend in your knee even when your leg is fully extended. If your saddle is too high, you might even be having some lower back pain from rocking your hips to help your legs at their full extension reach the pedals.

The Suspect: Saddle Too High

The Fix: Lower your saddle. At full extension, you want a slight bend in your knee (about 25 to 35 degrees) when the ball of your foot is placed on the pedal next to the pedal arm.

Sides of Knee Pain

If you use clipless pedals and have inner or outer knee pain only when you ride, this may be caused by knee/leg/foot alignment. Is your foot parallel to your bike frame, do you toe in, or are your heels pointing in? Are your knees bowed out or bowed in? Foot and knee position may be correctible – or it may be a function of your body mechanics.

If you use clip-in pedals, this source of your pain may be inaccurate alignment of your cleats mounted on your shoes. There are three directional factors to consider when mounting a cleat to your shoe: position along length of your foot, width of foot, and toe to heel direction.

The Suspect: Incorrect Foot Alignment or Incorrect Cleat Alignment

The Fixes:

- Barring any bio-mechanical issues, the lengths of your feet are roughly parallel to your bike frame and your knees are aligned with your feet.
- Cleat Position: Length of foot: Most people want the cleat mounted so the widest part of your foot is positioned next to where the pedal connects to the pedal arm.
- Cleat Position: Width of foot: Some shoes allow for a little adjustment side to side on the foot. Rule of thumb is to keep it neutral and place it to the center of your option.
- Cleat Position: Toe to Heel Direction: align the cleat so if you drew a line from the center of the shoe toe to the center

of the heel, you would cross through the center of the top and bottom of the cleat.

- Foot Alignment: Your foot may need support within your shoe or between your shoe and pedal. You may need an arch support, forefoot wedge, or even shims between your shoes and pedals. Analyzing foot in shoe and shoe on pedal takes expertise, and for this I recommend a professional bike fit.
- All of that said, I advocate pedals with "float" (cleats allowing for limited rotational movement) for anyone with knee problems. This allows your foot to find its natural position while accommodating your knee conditions.

Why do my Knees Hurt? The Common Reasons

Knee pain is one of the most common complaints in doctor visits. If you have ongoing knee pain off the bike, you may have something else going on with your knees. Some injuries require surgery, others need time to heal, and certain ones you just live with. Please see your doctor and get checked out. Common signs of knee injury are pain, swelling, and the knee catching, locking, or giving away.

I've listed some of the common knee complaints for general description purposes (2014)[6]. This is not meant to be a diagnostic tool. Please see your doctor if you suspect a knee injury.

Ligament Tear

The Anterior Cruciate Ligament (ACL) and Medial Collateral Ligament (MCL) are the most common ligament tears and cause instability in the knee. ACL (ACL is a stabilizer ligament on the inside of your knee) tears are commonly found in athletes who participate in high movement sports where they change direction rapidly (such as basketball, football, and soccer).

---

[6] OrthoInfo (2014) Common Knee Injuries. Retrieved on 8/26/15 from **http://orthoinfo.aaos.org/topic.cfm?topic=a00325**

The MCL (located on the side of your knee on the inside) is connected to your medial meniscus and so injury to the MCL may also involve your meniscus cartilage. Damage to the MCL often occurs from a direct impact to the outside of the knee pushing the knee sideways. Conversely, a direct blow to the inside of the knee may damage the ligament on the opposite side, the Lateral Collateral Ligament (LCL).

Inside your knee, attached behind the ACL, the Posterior Cruciate Ligament (PCL) may suffer injury from a direct impact to the front of the upper tibia while the knee is flexed. PCL damage often occurs from sports related motor vehicle accidents.

Your quadriceps muscles are connected by the quadriceps tendon to your patella (kneecap) which is connected by the patellar ligament to the tibia. Both the quadriceps tendon and patellar tendon can be strained (stretched or twisted and cause pain) or torn. This type of injury is more commonly seen among middle-aged people resulting from a hyper-flexion or jumping and landing awkwardly.

Cartilage Tear

There are two types of cartilage in your joint. Your articular cartilage is the shock-absorbing coating keeping your bones from rubbing together. The menisci are the tough fibrocartilage cushions around the periphery of the joint lying between your femur and tibia. Tears to your menisci often occur from sports or everyday living with moves involving twisting, quick changes of direction, pivoting, or a direct blow.

Chondromalacia Patella is damage to cartilage under the kneecap. A healthy patella glides up and down along the groove at the end of the femur. Damaged cartilage under the patella may be removed. The bone may be scraped to stimulate the cartilage healing.

Fractures

The kneecap is the most common broken bone in the knee, although the ends of the tibia and femur where they form the knee joint can also suffer from fracture. A fracture is often caused by a high impact trauma such as a car accident or fall from a high place.

Dislocation

Dislocation occurs when one or more of the bones in your knee are completely out of place. A subluxation is when the bones are partially out of place. Both can be caused by trauma or loose ligaments between the tibia and femur or around the patella. In people with normal knee structure, a dislocation is usually caused by a high-impact force such as car accident, sports injury, or a fall.

Arthritis

Arthritis has several forms of inflammatory or degenerative diseases affecting joints. The two most prevalent are discussed here. Each form presents symptoms in the same way: joint swelling, stiffness, and pain. It is the most prevalent crippling disease in the United States (2013)[7] (2014)[8]

Osteoarthritis

The most common form of joint disease is Osteoarthritis (OA) and it is among the top ten causes of disability in the world (2008)[9]. OA is a whole joint disease with a hallmark of cartilage destruction and

---

7   McKinley, Michael P., O'Loughlin Valerie Dean, and Bidle, Theresa Stouter (2013) *Anatomy & Physiology, An Integrative Approach*, New York, New York. McGraw-Hill.

8   National Institute of Arthritis and Musculoskeletal and Skin Diseases (2014), What is Rheumatoid Arthritis? Fast Facts: An Easy-to-Read Series of Publications for the Public, retrieved from **http://www.niams.nih.gov/Health_Info/Rheumatic_Disease/rheumatoid_arthritis_ff.asp#a**

9   National Collaborating Centre for Chronic Conditions (UK)Osteoarthritis: National clinical guideline for care and management in adults. London: Royal College of Physicians (UK); 2008. Retrieved on 8/27/15 from **http://www.ncbi.nlm.nih.gov/pubmed/?term=ational+Collaborating+Centre+for+Ch ronic+Conditions+(UK)Osteoarthritis%3A+National+clinical+guideline+for+care+and+manageme nt+in+adults.+London%3A+Royal+College+of+Physicians+(UK)%3B+2008.**

bone "remodeling" (thickening, bone collapse, bone spurs) followed by inflammation to mediate the degenerative conditions.

This wear-and-tear, chronic degenerative joint condition results when articular cartilage has worn down to allow bone to rub on bone. Removing the meniscus can accelerate the process due to less surface area available for weight bearing. As your weight bearing cartilage thins, changes occur such as growth of bone spurs and hardening of the bone (less shock absorbency of bone itself). Both result in pain.

Bone spurs (osteophytes) are bony outgrowths usually along the edge of a bone. They may inhibit mechanical motion of the knee, contributing to a limited range of motion or snapping or popping as a tendon or ligament rolls over the osteophyte. In addition to cartilage and bone degeneration, OA may also involve degeneration of ligaments and hypertrophy (enlargement) of the joint capsule.

Rheumatoid Arthritis

Rheumatoid Arthritis is an autoimmune disorder where an individual's immune system attacks their own tissues. It is most prevalent in women, with onset in middle age (40-50 years old). In addition to typical arthritis symptoms of joint swelling and pain, rheumatoid arthritis also may involve muscle weakness, osteoporosis, and assorted problems with both blood vessels and the heart.

Rheumatoid arthritis starts with inflammation of the synovial membrane in joints. Every moving joint essentially has a sack of lubricating synovial fluid. When inflamed, the outside of this sack (the membrane) can allow fluid and white blood cells to leak from small blood vessels into the joint cavity, resulting in an increase of synovial fluid volume. This makes the joint swell and the inflamed synovial membrane thickens. The articular cartilage on the ends of bones wears off and the underlying bone becomes eroded. Ligaments and tendons may rupture causing greater deformity.

"They Just Hurt", Snap, Crack, and Pop

It is common to hear your joints crack or pop when you go through the range of motion, especially your knees. (2015)[10]. If there is no associated pain or swelling, there may be no cause for alarm. The snaps and pops may be from the articular or meniscal cartilage having a little rough spot, small divot, or uneven area. When the rough spots rollover each other, they can make noises. It could also be sounds coming from your ligaments which tighten and stretch as you move. If there is pain involved, you should certainly have it checked out by a doctor.

Your knee is the hardest-working joint in your body. You might be tempted to just give in to the aching and quit everything. But since you picked up this book, I think you want something more. Perhaps you want to reduce your pain and make your knees feel better. It could be you are ready to make your knees stronger. Maybe you want to become more active and need to know how while still doing good for your knees. Or you might be recovering from a knee surgery and want a smart course of action following your physical therapy. Healthy Knees Cycling can help!

Of all the activities I've tried over the past 25 + years since I quit running and downhill skiing, riding a bike has been, by far, the most fun and the best for my knees. I often joke I'm no longer a biped, but instead a two-wheeled human. My knees actually feel better on a bike than when walking around.

Why is cycling so good for your knees? That is our book's next chapter and could be yours as well.

---

[10] O'Neill Hill, L. and Kercher MD, J. (2015) *What is Your Knee Telling You.*
Web MD Knee Pain Health Center. Retrieved 8/24/15 from
http://www.webmd.com/pain-management/knee-pain/features/knee-cracks-pops

CHAPTER 2

WHY CYCLING IS SO GOOD FOR YOUR KNEES

I get it. When your knees hurt, you don't feel much like moving around. It's like someone took your knees and replaced them with squeaky, rusty, painful, hard to move hinges. I've been there. It feels bad. It is hard to see past the pain and discomfort. But here's the thing: when you use movement that is good for your knees, you are nourishing them. It's like oiling your knee joints and they start to feel better and move better. The "oil" I use for my knees is bicycling and I want to share WHY it is so good for your knees before we get to the HOW.

Cycling Not Only Helps Your Knees, it nourishes your ankles and hips and can help with weight management.

Cycling is Fun! Feel Healthy, Active, and Enjoy Life!

Think back to when you first learned how to ride a bike. Remember the feeling of freedom? The excitement of adventure? The feeling of accomplishment? You can have this again AND you are doing good things for your knees! Riding a bike, whether indoors or outside, might bring back the joy of living. As your knees get stronger, you'll feel healthier, become more active, and get more out of life.

Cycling Strengthens Your Joints

You can have a variety of things wrong with your knee (torn ligament, missing cartilage, arthritis), but you can make it stronger. Your knee is stabilized by ligaments holding the bones in place. Your muscles attach to bones by tendons and also add to your joint stability. During each pedal stroke, there are varying stresses in compression and expansion within the knee joint that help ligaments and tendons become stronger. This gives you more stability.

Your hip flexor and extensor muscles play an important role in cycling and strengthen your hip joint as well. The gentle movement through your ankle also activates your foot extension and flexion muscles, serving to strengthen your ankle as well.

The Troika of Goodness for your Knees: No Impact, No Weight Bearing, No Lateral Movement

Your goal is knee movement without irritation, right? Cycling is perfect for knees, hips, and ankles!

No Impact

Cycling is a non-impact activity. What does this mean, exactly. Consider: each time you take a step while walking (or running), your heel strike – along with your ankle, knee, and hip joints – absorb the force of your body weight *plus* effects of gravity. Each time your foot hits the ground when you're running, it can impart a force up to 2.5 times your body weight[11]. This force is absorbed by your joints. The knee catches the largest portion since it has the greatest movement.

Cycling, along with activities like swimming or using an elliptical machine, are considered to be "no-impact" since there is no repeated foot strike with the ground. There will be some compression in the joints caused by the movements, but the percussive heel strike has been removed. This is good, especially for arthritic joints.

---

11 Keller, TS, Weisberger AM, Ray JL, et al (1996) *Relationship between vertical ground reaction force and speed during walking, slow jogging, and running.* PubMed.gov. Retrieved on 11/14/15 from **http://www.ncbi.nlm.nih.gov/pubmed/11415629**

Every time you have an impact-caused compression, the bones in your knees come closer together. If your knee joint is healthy, this impact is no problem because your cartilage is doing its job of absorbing shock. However, if you are missing cartilage, have arthritic changes in your knee, or have an issue with your ligaments or tendons, impact activities may cause more wear-and-tear in the joint.

No Weight Bearing

Why is cycling considered no weight bearing? The seat is holding most of your weight. Think of the difference with an elliptical machine, where you are still standing and bearing your weight in your feet. On a bike, your weight is in your butt on the saddle. You could completely take your feet off your pedals and you won't fall down. With cycling, you get the movement in your ankles, knees, and hips, without the weight of your entire body stressing your joints.

But wait, it gets even better…

No Lateral Movement

Lateral movement refers to side-to-side movement of your knees, such as downhill skiing or shuffle steps in basketball. Lateral movement is the source of much knee damage and pain. There is practically NO lateral knee movement on a bike. The straight forward knee path of pedaling keeps your knees in good alignment without any of the potentially irritating side-to-side movement.

Strengthens the Muscles Supporting Your Joint

While your knee joint is held together by its ligaments, it is also stabilized and controlled by its muscles with their tendons. As you use your muscles, they get stronger and their attachments (tendons) to the bones do, too. As you perform movement and strengthening exercises, the muscle tendon pulls on the bone which also makes the bone stronger.

Stronger muscles, stronger bones, and more stable ankle, knees, and hips = win-win-win!

Non-Impact Movement Stimulates Healthy Joint Fluid and helps Reduce Pain

Your ankle, knee, and hip joints are made for movement. Movement stimulates the joint to keep producing your healthy joint fluid. This thick, slippery synovial fluid acts as a lubricant for movement, nourishment for cartilage, and helps to cushion the joint structures[12] and reduce inflammation.

When you use your knees in a healthy way through cycling, you'll have fun along the way and do a world of good for your knees. You'll also gain knee stability, reduce the joint aggravating stresses of impact from other activities, improve your knee and leg strength, and reduce pain. Doesn't that sound great? I bet you want to know how to get going! Let's explore all the ways you can ride.

Matthew Iwersen, Tennis Pro, has loved tennis all his life. He played for a D1 college and went on to work in the field as a tennis teaching professional. Matt's 50-year love of tennis also created wear and tear on his ankles. When his arthritic pain was the worst (prior to having an ankle replaced) he said "Cycling is one of the ways I can get my heart rate up and sooth my ankle at the same time." Matt has since had his ankle replaced and still uses indoor cycling as his primary cardio workout.
"I don't want to chew up my new ankle by over doing it on the tennis court. So I cycle and I love how I feel when I am done. No ankle pain and a great workout."

---

[12] Holland, K (2015) *Understanding Cartilage, Joints, and the Aging Process.* Healthline. Retrieved on 9/16/15 from: **http://www.healthline.com/health/osteoarthritis/understanding-aging-and-joints**

CHAPTER 3

CYCLING OPTIONS...
THERE ARE MANY WAYS!

The best thing about riding a bike is: there are so many different ways to do it. The most important thing is to *start*. It may be simpler, at first, to ride a stationary bike inside (I talk about this in later chapters) with guidance from a Healthy Knees coach or by following the workouts included in this book. You may find it's your favorite way to ride. However, I've known many people who start out on an indoor bike and enjoy it so much they buy a bike to ride outside. Before you know it, they are preparing for a charity bike ride or planning a cycling adventure with their kids or grandkids. Cycling with a group is a wonderful way to meet new people who share an interest with you. Whether you are inside or outside, here are some ideas about how to get rolling.

If you are already a cyclist, you may want to skip this chapter. But you don't have to be a bike racer to enjoy riding a bike. There are so many ways to use a bike – from around your neighborhood to around the world - and all of them can help your knees (as long as you follow the four Healthy Knees Fundamentals!)

Target Training (inside or outside)

Use cycling to get stronger whether you are inside on a stationary bike or outdoors. In addition to strengthening your knees, you can use cycling intervals to improve your cardiovascular endurance and improve your lung capacity. Riding indoors is a great time focus on technique since you do not have the outdoor distractions of traffic, stop signs, potholes, rain, wind, dogs, etc. You can focus on pedal stroke, pedal speed, muscle power, muscle and cardio endurance, and even hill climbing by building the muscle strength and coordination to pedal while standing on your pedals.

Recreational Rides

Riding a bike is just plain fun. Start small – even if it's just once around your block – and grow from there. Gain skills and confidence on your bike as you begin to explore your neighborhood, visit your county parks, ride some trails, and make the trip to the grocery store on your bike! Help the world a little bit by riding your bike more and using a car less. Not only is it good for you, but good for the environment.

Social Cycling with a Bike Club

Join your local bike club and meet new people. Many clubs have organized rides for all levels of riders from the beginners learning how to ride in a group or a Tuesday morning "coffee" ride. Some bicycle clubs offer day-long multi-mile rides or training rides where you have the opportunity to ride harder, get faster, and show your stuff.

Events and/or Competition

There are plenty of opportunities to ride your bike in fundraiser events, endurance events, multi-sport relays (each person on the team does a different sport) or competition (e.g. triathlon either as an individual or a team), or straight out bicycle racing. Setting a goal for yourself for such an event gives your training a purpose. Working with a coach to develop a training plan is also a good idea. Find a cause you believe in and sign up for their bicycle event so you can train with a purpose! Help others while you help yourself.

"I started the healthy knees camp w/chronic knee cap arthritis pain - by the fifth week of camp the pain has gone from a level of 'very frequent' to almost "non-existent". I also have a chronic back issue resulting in sciatica down one leg and the well-crafted stationary bike work-out has proven to be excellent for relief."

Deborah D.

Destination or Adventure Travel

My favorite way to travel is by bicycle because you go fast enough to get somewhere but are on the backroads where you hear and see so much more than if you are in a car or on a train. You have the opportunity to meet people, stop in the small towns, and pause when something piques your interest. You are out in the elements (sometimes for better or worse) to feel and hear all around you. Plus the bonus: you can more fully enjoy eating the local fare when you've burned all those calories riding your bike during the day.

"My favorite memory on our Danube cycle trip with our extended family (including grandchildren) was a day it was raining. We all loved the feeling of being in the weather outdoors with the fresh, warm rain on our faces."

Walt L., age 81

There are many ways to travel by bike and options for how far you ride each day:

- Fully supported tour with a guide: The tour company guide leads the ride each day, the company carries your gear for you, and – depending on your tour – you may sleep in hotels or camp. You don't worry about a thing, your itinerary is set, and you get fully pampered! There is usually an option to "get a lift" if you aren't feeling up to some or the entire ride for the day.

- Semi-Supported Tour: The tour company transports your gear from hotel to hotel (or campground to campground) on a planned route, but you ride on your own. You enjoy the freedom of riding your bike, taking a side trip if you wish, and stopping when you want.
- On your Own: You carry your own gear and plan your own trip. The ultimate in freedom! You can choose if you'll go lighter and sleep in hotels or go fully packed by carrying your own cooking utensils, sleeping bag, and tent. The more gear you carry, the slower you'll ride and the fewer the miles you can make each day. But this is about the journey, right? There is a certain satisfaction and confidence that comes with being self-contained.

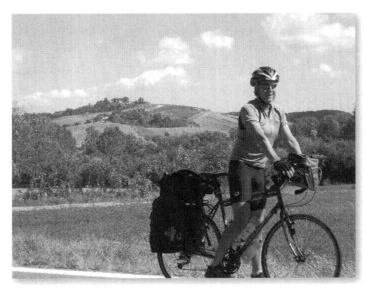

The point is to get on a bike. You definitely want to follow the Healthy Knees Foundations (later in this book), setting yourself up for success. Now that you are excited about getting on a bike, let's get going!

CHAPTER 4

GET READY TO RIDE

This stage discusses the nuts-and-bolts of having fun on a bike (if you are an experienced cyclist, you could probably skim this chapter.)

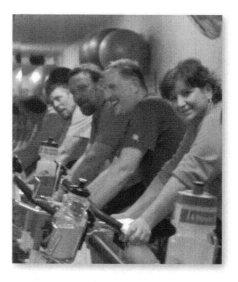

The first step is to choose where you want to ride: inside or outside. If you are using a bike at a health club, I talk about the general varieties found there. If you are thinking about buying a bike, I give a brief overview of bikes types to familiarize you with the array of choices. For those who already own a bike, I share ways you can turn it into a stationary bike so you can do some focused riding inside at home. Of course, we must talk about what to wear so you'll feel comfortable while you ride. Getting ready to ride is not just about your bike and your clothes, but also how you prepare your body with fuel. What and when do you eat before, during, and after you exercise. This section gives you everything you need to know about getting ready to ride.

Choose Indoor or Outdoor - or Both!

When I talk about indoor cycling to some of my bike friends, I sometimes hear, "I only ride outside," followed by a snarky comment or haughty look that generally insinuates I am nuts for riding inside.

While I also love riding outside, I find my indoor training gives me consistency, focus, strength, and a solid base for my outdoor adventures. Here is my comparison of indoor vs. outdoor cycling:

Indoor Benefits

Indoor Cycling is Convenient!

The weather is always perfect for an indoor ride. It is easy to hop on a spinning bike (or your own bike on a trainer) and go. No worries about rain, traffic, temperature, wind, potholes, cars, or dogs. Bam! You get a great workout done in 30 to 90 minutes.

Great for Beginners: You Don't Have to Worry About How Well (or not) You Can Ride a Bike.

Stationary bikes are…stationary! You don't worry about tipping over or steering in a straight line. It is simple! Just get on the bike and pedal.

You Can Control It

You are in control of how hard you ride. You control your intensity by choosing how much tension to add or by selecting an easier or harder gear. If you want to back off your intensity, you can. If you want to increase it, you can. You can get the most out of your workout, every day.

Heart Rate Training

Your heart is the most important muscle in your body, yet most people overlook specific training for the heart. It is more important than six-pack abs!

Indoors, you can be very specific about your level of effort. You don't worry about the terrain, cars, or stopping for lights that can interrupt your interval or change your intensity.

Focusing on heart rate training helps your heart become stronger and more resilient. You can see improvements in resting heart rate, heart rate recovery, and heart rate threshold (aerobic/anaerobic capacity). All three are important for heart health. I discuss this more, later.

And no, just going hard all of the time is NOT usually the best thing for your heart. Good indoor cycling programs (like Healthy Knees or Cycle Moles!) focus on a variety of efforts through interval training with a plan.

Calorie Burn: Easier or Harder than Outdoors?

We love that cycling burns a lot of calories! A typical 150-pound person burns about 500 calories in a 60-minute class.

Is it easier or harder than outdoors? That depends on how you ride your bike outside. *Most recreational cyclists find it harder to reach the level of intensity or heart rate outside they consistently achieve while inside.*

Indoors, there is no coasting. You are constantly working throughout your ride. It is a common belief that an indoor effort has more intensity (and caloric burn) than an outdoor ride. This may be especially true for most recreational cyclists because your intensity level is usually higher when you are working indoors than when you go for an outdoor ride. Competitive athletes who have a training plan for their outdoor rides can achieve high calorie burn efforts indoors or out. You can certainly measure this with your heart rate monitor and compare the calories burned for 60 minutes indoor vs. 60 minutes outside.

Focused Workout and Specific Training

In many indoor cycling classes, you'll find a random assortment of workouts providing some health benefit and keeping your heart rate at around 75 to 95 percent of your maximum rate – the suggested range according to the American Council on Exercise – and a high calorie burn.

I love that Healthy Knees and Cycle Moles workouts have a plan with every workout aiming for a specific benefit: building your foundation skills, aerobic base, speed work, hill climbing, improving your metabolism, and so on. This kind of focus is harder to attain outside.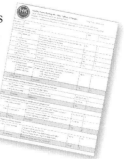

Hamstrings Get Extra Attention

Most spinning bikes have a fly-wheel which is a 30- to 40-pound fixed-gear wheel providing much of the rotational resistance as you pedal. There is no coasting on a spinning bike since the weighted wheel keeps the pedals moving like a fixed-gear bike.

This is both good and bad.

Good because your hamstrings must work harder to slow down the pedals if you are slowing your speed. This is different from riding outdoors where you are pedaling against the friction of the road, plus wind resistance, which requires more work from your quadriceps and hip flexors.

Bad because you can let the wheel do some of the work for you. When you get the wheel spinning, the momentum pushes your pedals a little bit.

Social Fun in a Group

It's a little hard to be social outdoors because you normally ride single file to be safe; plus the wind and road noise makes it hard to hear each other.

With indoor cycling, you have the camaraderie of your group (you are all in this together!), instructions by your coach (so you don't even need to think about what comes next), great music, and the support and enthusiasm of everyone around you.

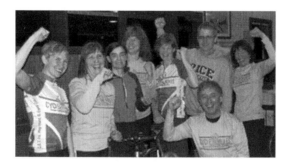

Outdoor Benefits

Its Outdoors (Good and Bad)

It is hard to beat riding in great weather with fresh air on country roads or on forest trails.

I love riding my bike outside more than just about anything else. I live in a place where, within 10 minutes, I can ride my road bike on quiet country roads or my mountain bike on some of the world's best cross country trails. I love putting my bags on my bike and heading out for travel. In 1990 I spent 10 months traveling around the world on my bike with my husband. I think there is no better way to see your hometown and the world than on a bike.

That said, though, there are always things to deal with: traffic, rude drivers, stoplights, dogs, poor weather, darkness, temperature, food, water, getting lost (which can be a good thing), flats, and other mechanical issues.

You Can't Control It

Unlike your ride inside, you can't control everything about your outdoor ride. Of course, you can pick your route; but there are plenty of variables along the way. When you get to a hill, you climb the hill. When you are on the flats with a headwind, you power through. If it starts raining, you deal with it. You need to be ready for everything and this makes life exciting.

Hills are Different

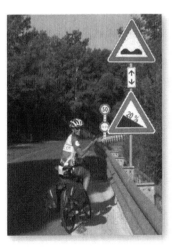

Riding a hill outdoors is different than indoors no matter how much you prepare for it inside. For one thing, outdoors the bike moves under you instead of you moving over the stationary bike. This movement is nice because, if you are standing, you can pull the handlebars to help you leverage more power and keep your body relatively still while your bike rocks side to side.

Also, your body position on your bike changes based on the grade of the hill. The steeper the hill, the more forward your position.

Finally, the hill ends when the hill ends, not when you want to ease up (that you can sneakily do in a cycling class).

Thrill of the Unknown: Risks and Beauty

Every ride can bring something new around the corner. This is what I love about bicycling outside! You need to stay aware, be in the moment, and keep your senses active. This is also why I never recommend listening to music while you ride – instead, use your ears to help you stay aware of risks and hear the beauty of the great outdoors such as bird song, kids laughing, and secret waterfalls.

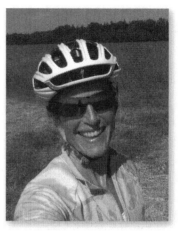

Note: Always, always, ALWAYS wear your helmet. I know many people who would not be with us today if it weren't for the protection provided by their helmets. Me included.

Ride Inside: Stationary Bike Options

To improve your knee health through cycling....you'll need a bike! You have two general options: stationary bike (indoor cycling bikes aka "Spinning®" bikes, or "club" bikes), or your own bike mounted on a trainer.

Indoor Cycling Bikes

Stationary bikes come in two general categories; "spinning®" bikes or "club" bikes.

The stationary indoor cycling bike or Spinning® bike is a simple bike without pre-determined programs. You are in charge of how hard or how easy it is to pedal based on how much tension or resistance you add through turning a knob or shifting the gear.

Here are a few common types of bikes used in indoor cycling classes. Spinning® and the "Spinner®" bike are trademarked names created Mad Dogg Athletics. But the term "spinning" has become synonymous with any stationary indoor cycle.

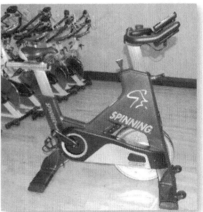

Yellow bike: Lemond RevMaster with belt drive; Grey bike Star Trac Spinning bike with chain drive; Black with red Keiser M3i with Magnetic resistance.

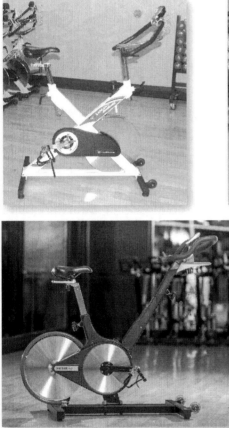

There are generally four types of indoor cycling bikes and many, many brands: wind trainer (with a fan), belt drive, chain drive, and magnetic resistance. As with outdoor bikes, the geometry of the indoor bike varies from brand to brand. This means one frame and geometry may fit you better than others, especially if you are very tall or very short.

Three adjustments I watch for healthy knees:

1) Distance between Pedals

This distance cannot usually be changed on a bike. This plays into the comfort of your knees. I find pedals set closer together, mimicking an outdoor bike, feel better on knees. This has to do with the "Q angle" – the relationship of your hip crest, thigh bone, and knee. Women tend to have a larger Q angle than do men. Many club bikes seem to have their pedals set a little wider apart.

2) Adjustable Handlebars, Fore/Aft

Pretty much all bikes let you adjust the handlebars up and down. But some bikes do not let you move the handlebars closer to or farther away from the saddle. This means a short person likely overextends to reach the handlebars, or moves the saddle closer to the handlebars than they should for good alignment with the knees. This can cause discomfort in arms, shoulders, lower back, and/or front of the knees. A very tall person will be crunched or have to set the seat so far back their legs are out of alignment.

3) Adjustable Saddle, Fore/Aft

Most bikes allow you to adjust the saddle up and down, but some may not allow you to move the saddle closer to or farther away from the handlebars. The ability to move your seat so your knees are properly aligned with your feet is key to knee happiness. Do NOT ride a bike that puts your knee in a poor position (more details on this in "Healthy Knees Fundamentals")

"Club" Stationary Bikes

A club bike is a stationary bike with pre-set programs and usually a monitor to display your progress. If you choose a program, it automatically adjusts how hard or how easy it is to pedal. To create your own workout, there is almost always a manual option. You can increase or decrease resistance (how hard or how easy it is to pedal) as you wish. These bikes are usually in the cardio area of a gym mixed in with the elliptical machines and treadmills.

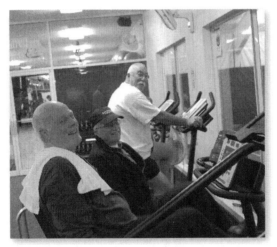

Let's say you want to do your own workout on one of the club bikes. You can either follow one of the programs on the bikes or, by switching to manual, follow your own program (such as a Healthy Knees workout in this book or perhaps a Cycle Moles program you've downloaded from the internet).

Club bikes sometimes have a wider distance between the pedals than indoor cycling bikes. If you are set up properly but still feel pain (especially on the inside or outside of your knee), this wider distance could be the culprit. You may need to switch to an indoor cycle bike for more comfort.

Your own Bike on a Trainer

Most people don't own their own spinning-style bike, so what can you do if you want indoor workouts at home?

Turn your bicycle into a stationary bike with specially-built "trainers."

A trainer usually hooks to the rear wheel axel and then, when you sit on the bike and pedal, a roller on the rear tire creates resistance. Trainers come in a variety of models and are priced from under $100 to more than $900 depending on the features you desire.

There are generally three types of resistance trainers: resistance is created by fan, magnet, or fluid. A fan trainer is the loudest and uses wind to create the resistance. Magnetic trainers are quieter than the fan and use the more powerful magnetic resistance. Fluid trainers are the quietest of all and have a magnetic flywheel with fluid chambers for the smoothest resistance. Trainers hold your bike in one rigid position and are great for overall training, including strength and power intervals against the resistance.

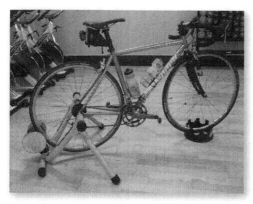

Bike on Kurt Kinetic Trainer Rear View

A fourth option for a stationary trainer is "rollers." Your bike is not attached, but instead the wheels sit upon three cylinders and you balance as you ride. When you first try this, it feels like your bike is on an ice rink. As you are learning, I suggest you set your rollers in a doorway. When you fall (and you will!), you'll catch yourself in the door frame. With practice, you gain confidence and balance. Rollers allow a little more natural movement of the bike and are great for improving your overall body balance and pedal technique.

Ride Outside: Your Choices

It's not just one type of bike anymore! There are bicycles to fit every comfort level and style of riding you can imagine. Prices start in the $100s and can reach over $10,000 (gasp!). I suggest you ride several styles and brands of bikes and make the investment for one with good, durable, and replaceable parts. Most bicycle stores have a variety of models and price ranges. When you are comfortable on your bike, you will ride it. If you are not, you won't. It is that simple.

I highly suggest working with your local bike stores to compare different models. This lets you discover what you like best.

Here are some questions to help determine what kind of bike to buy:

- Where do you like to ride? (roads, trails, or both)
- What kind of riding experience do you have (new to cycling or experienced cyclist)?
- How far do you like to ride?
- How often do you want to ride?
- Have you had a bike in the past you liked or disliked? Why?
- Who do you want to ride with? What do they ride?

The following is a very brief synopsis of bicycle categories. Each category has many variations and price ranges to go with it. For healthy knees, I recommend a bike with many gears (especially for climbing hills). Keep in mind you can always change the saddle on a bike to match your comfort level, but your body position is determined by the geometry of the bike. If you want to sit up more, choose a hybrid bike. If you want speed on the road, a road or touring bike is for you. If you are looking to explore off-road trails, consider a mountain bike.

Hybrid or City Bike

The hybrid or city bike provides the advantages of both mountain and road bike. They usually have a more padded seat, medium width tires, and upright handlebars for a comfortable more upright position on roads, bike paths, and non-technical paved or unpaved trails.

Mountain Bike

Mountain bikes are designed for off-road trails, have low gears for hill-climbing, and generally have a less-padded seat, wide knobby tires and flat handlebars. Depending on your preference, you can buy a mountain bike that has no suspension, just front suspension, or full suspension.

Road Bike

Road bikes are made for speed on smooth pavement. They have narrow saddles, smooth skinny tires, and "drop" handlebars. Road bikes are usually lighter weight than other bicycles and are not usually equipped to carry a load. The geometry on a road bike has your body leaned forward toward the handlebars.

Touring Bike/Cyclo-cross

Touring and cyclo-cross bikes usually have a longer wheel base than a road bike and are more durable and heavier. Tires can be wider and either smooth or with light tread. These bikes usually have brackets to mount a rear or front rack for carrying a load (or touring gear). The body position is similar to the road bike with a lean forward toward the drop handlebars. If you are thinking of an adventure cyclo road tour and carrying your own gear, this is the bike for you.

Specialty Bikes

So many bikes! This is not an exhaustive list, but an idea of alternatives to the main four categories listed above. In addition, there are single speeds, unicycles, tricycles, and all of the bikes falling somewhere in between.

a. **Cruiser** – Single speed (maybe 3-speed), coaster brakes, and designed for comfort riding.

b. **Time Trial/Triathlon** – specialty road bikes with a design that maximizes aerodynamic flow to minimize wind resistance against your body with the most aggressive laid forward body position.

c. **Recumbent Bikes** – have a full sized seat (more like a chair) with a back rest offering a laid back position. Recumbent bikes have two or three wheels. The design of a recumbent puts you closer to the ground with your legs and feet in front of (rather than below) your torso. While a recumbent may be more comfortable on your hind end, they are more challenging to ride up a hill. Make sure you love the geometry of the bike and feel of the riding position.

d. **Electric Assist**

Electric assist bikes are gaining in popularity in the United States. They come in all styles: Cruiser, Hybrid, Road, Mountain, and even folding models. Electric bikes have an integrated electric motor to boost your pedal power (very handy for going up hills!). The added weight of the motor makes these bikes heavier than their non-motorized counterparts.

What to Wear

The three most important parts of what you wear cycling are your helmet, clothes and your shoes. Your clothing depends, in part, on if you are riding inside on a stationary bike or outside.

When riding inside, you are not moving through the air to cool you and you tend to get sweatier (sweat is good!). Wear layers with a sweat-wicking top. You'll still want the padded shorts!

When riding outside, you must dress according to the weather. Is it hot or cold? Is it sunny or rainy? Do you need a wind jacket? How do you prepare for unexpected weather changes?

Everything but the Shoe

You want to wear clothes that are comfortable to sweat in and won't bind or constrict movement. Your hind end may be of most concern while on a bike, so let's start there.

Bottoms: Bike Shorts

Bicycle shorts have a padded crotch for a very good reason. The padding or "chamois" (or "shammy") helps protect your sensitive areas and gives you greater comfort. And some chamois help keep bacteria from flourishing when you are wearing your bike shorts for a long time – like a full day's ride. Be sure to wash your bike shorts after every ride; I let mine air dry to help the fabric last longer.

If you don't have bike shorts or are not yet ready to invest in them, wear a pair of snug fitting shorts or athletic pants that won't bind up around your legs or crotch. Binding causes rubbing, which leads to discomfort and pain.

Travel Tip: If you are traveling and need to wash your shorts, the chamois can take a while to dry. Try this tip: After washing, lay your shorts on a towel and roll the towel up tightly. Twist the towel and stomp on it. Twist it the other way and stomp on it again. Voila! You've just taken out about 70% of the moisture. Your shorts will probably dry while hanging overnight.

*See the video: **www.healthykneesbook.com/resources***

Sweat-Wicking Shirt + Layers

Wearing a bike jersey or sweat-wicking top helps regulate your body temperature, so you won't get chilled from a sweaty cotton shirt sticking to you. How much or little coverage you want is up to you. When riding inside, an outer layer, such as a light athletic jacket or sweatshirt may make it more comfortable for you during your warmup or cool down. I tend to sweat a lot, so I like to put on a sweatshirt during my cool down so I won't get chilled. Wool riding jerseys are terrific for cool to cold weather.

More: Other Apparel You'll Need Outside

- Bike gloves to pad and protect your hands

  Bike gloves have multiple functions. First and foremost is to protect your hands if you were to fall or if you are trail riding through snaggy, shrubby areas. Pavement or trails can be very rough on skin. Second is to give a little more cushion to your palms for gripping your handlebars. Third is to keep your hands warm if it is cool out or even to protect from sunburn.

- Helmet to protect your head

  Never ride without a helmet! Your helmet straps and headband must be adjusted properly for your helmet to do its job. The front of your helmet should be worn low on your forehead; the front and back straps meeting just below your earlobe and tightened to allow about one finger to slip between the strap and your jaw. I've been known to go up to complete strangers and ask if I may adjust their helmet. It is easy to do and you'll need to adjust your own every few months to keep it in the correct position to protect your head.

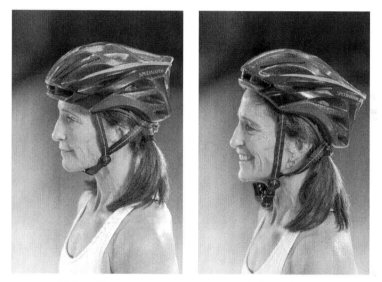

Helmet Correct   Helmet Wrong

- Windcoat or Raincoat

    Riding in inclement weather is much more enjoyable when you have the appropriate gear. When the weather looks iffy, roll up your coat and carry it in your jersey pocket, just in case.

- Leg protection if it is cool/cold (full tights or knee warmers)

    Full length, calf length, and knee length tights are available with or without the chamois. I prefer no chamois, but wear the tights over my bike shorts to give me an extra layer of warmth and protection.

- Toe Covers or Booties over your shoes if it is cold

    Toe covers and booties are worth their weight in gold. I do not like cold toes! Another method for warm feet is to put a plastic bag over your sock before you slip on your shoe. While not very pretty, it is cheap and does help to hold heat (and sweat) in.

- Headband or skull cap under your helmet if it is cold

    Headbands and skull caps come in a variety of materials and thicknesses. I prefer a headband to keep my ears warm but let my head give off heat. If you tend to be cold, covering your head is one of the best ways to stay warm. If a headband or skull cap is not for you, you can try a helmet cover to hold in heat.

The Shoe Depends upon the Pedal

Flat Pedals

Any shoe can be used on a flat pedal, even a stiletto, but I don't recommend it for your workouts! On flat pedals you can really only push down (which means you are missing out on the other three parts of your pedal stroke – more on this in "Healthy Knees Secrets to Cycling").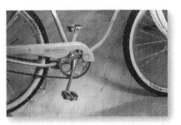

Toe Cages

Some pedals provide a cage for the toe of your foot to slip into so you can lightly bind your foot to the pedal with the pull of a strap. Toe cages help you get more power out of your pedal stroke because they give you some ability to pull back, lift up, and kick over the top as well as push down on your pedals.

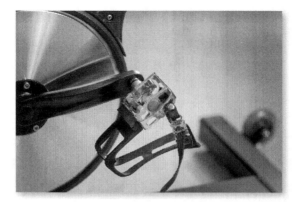

Cleats, Clipless, or Clip-in

Why the name confusion? Cleats, clipless, or clip-ins all refer to a pedal system where a cleat on your shoe locks into the pedal. They are called "clipless" because there is no toe-clip (or toe cage) even though there is a clip (or cleat) on the bottom of your shoe to attach your foot to the pedal. Goofy, I know.

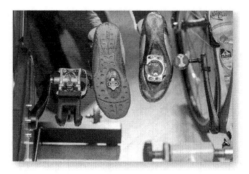

If you are in a cycling class, find out the brand of the clip-ins on the pedal. The most common on spin bikes are "SPD" compatible. If you want to wear bike shoes with cleats that lock into the pedal, they need to match the type on the bike pedal.

Many indoor cycles offer dual pedals with toe cages on one side and clip-in SPD pedals on the other. Most club bikes come with a simple strap to secure your foot to the pedal better than a flat pedal.

Float vs Fixed Pedals for Your Knees

If you are considering clipless pedals for your own bike, there are many choices. Pay close attention to "float". Float refers to the amount of rotational movement given to your shoe while clipped in to the pedal. Zero float means your foot is locked into one position – and if you have knee issues, more care needs to be given to correct alignment of the cleat to accommodate your knee and foot position or it may exacerbate your knee pain.

I recommend choosing a pedal which allows "float" or rotational movement of your shoe. I like this option for those with knee issues because it is much more forgiving and allows for rotational movement which you may need to accommodate your knee movement in your pedal stroke. It also means, as your knee feels better or worse and your alignment changes slightly, you don't need to tinker with the position of your cleat so much. Your foot can naturally fall into the most comfortable position.

And Now...The Shoe on your Pedal

For starters, any athletic shoe works. You can certainly ride with your sneakers, but you may find your feet get tired. This is because regular athletic shoes have a softer, flexible sole that allows your foot to flex. You may "feel" the imprint of the pedal through the sole to your foot, and you may feel tightness of the toe cage around the top of your foot.

For increased comfort, I prefer a bike shoe when riding indoors and out. Bike shoes, with or without cleats, have a <u>very stiff sole</u> which does three important things:

1) A stiff sole transfers more energy to your pedal because most of the force goes into the pedal and is not lost in movement of your foot;

2) A stiff sole is more comfortable because your foot is stable. Your foot won't get tired from flexing. If you've ever had issues with plantar fasciitis (inflammation of the tissue called the plantar fascia along the bottom of your foot) or foot cramping, you'll definitely want a stiff cycling shoe.

3) Some flat pedals have "teeth" for gripping shoes. The hard sole of a bike shoe protects your foot from feeling the impression of the "teeth" through your shoe.

Shoe (foot) Placement on the Pedal

Does it matter where your foot is on the pedal? You bet!

Place the widest part of your foot/shoe on the pedal right where the pedal connects to the pedal arm. This helps you transfer the most energy into your pedal. For those of you with smaller shoe sizes, you probably won't need to insert your foot all the way to the end of most toe cages.

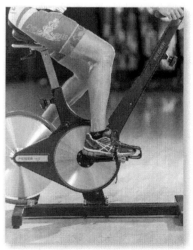

Same with your bike cleats. They should be positioned on your shoe so the widest part of your foot is next to where the pedal connects to the pedal arm.

Foot placement on the pedal is the place to start when getting a good fit on your bike. If your *foot* is in the wrong place, your *knees* are, too. This can cause all sorts of problems.

Fueling Your Ride

What, when, and how much you eat and drink affects the quality of your exercise time. Want to get the biggest benefit out of your time on a bike? Follow these simple rules.

Nutrition 101

The food we eat and beverages we drink provide the fuel we need to grow and sustain life. All food is digested and stored (or eliminated) by our bodies in three main nutrient categories: Carbohydrates, Lipids, and Proteins. Vitamins (organic nutrients) and minerals (inorganic nutrients) are important for bone formation, nerve and muscle function, and many chemical functions. Fiber is not digested but helps to move wastes through our digestive system. Don't forget water! Water makes up 2/3 of the body and acts as a biological solvent. The following chart is a VERY general summary.

Nutrient	Forms	Description	Function
Carbohydrates	Fruits Grains Vegetables Milk	Carbohydrate molecules contain glucose (sugars) and are available in simple to complex forms.	Glucose is stored as glycogen in muscles and liver for use as energy and for brain function.
Lipids	Saturated: animal fats – meats, butter, cheese Unsaturated: Olive oil, avocado, fish	Lipid molecules (fats) are insoluble in water and include oils, animal fats, waxes, and steroids. Fats are classified as saturated and unsaturated.	Fats are useful! Different types are stored for energy, compose all cell membranes, are in plasma membranes, serve as hormones… and more!
Proteins	Meats Fish Beans Rice Eggs and Dairy	A complete protein is made up of the 8 essential Amino Acids (the ones your body cannot produce) of 20 different amino acids.	Unlike glycogen and fats, proteins have no large storage depot and are used right away (or converted to fat for storage). Proteins are the primary building blocks for muscle, bone, skin, hair, enzyme structure, and more.

Fuel Before Exercise

With any type of workout, it's a good idea to take in some food prior to exercise. Here are some general guidelines (there are VOLUMES of books written about sports nutrition; this is very general information): If you eat a big meal, give yourself two hours before you exercise.

If you eat something light (banana, yogurt, or any easily digestible food), give yourself no fewer than 30 minutes. Some people feel they can exercise on an empty stomach. However, most find if they are smart about what and when they eat, food gives them greater energy for a better workout.

Whatever you decide works best for you, make sure you fuel your ride!

Fuel During Exercise

If you start to feel light headed or your energy runs out during exercise, you are probably low on fuel. It's time to eat or drink something with calories in it.

When planning to exercise for more than 60 minutes, you may need to take in some calories during your activity to replace those carbohydrates you use. What you eat has a lot to do with YOU. Find foods that sit well in your belly while you are exercising.

The quantity of calories you need/can process varies based on your body, type of activity you are doing, your intensity, and the weather (think 90 minutes high-intensity training ride on a very hot day vs. a casual-pace 100-mile century ride in cold weather). Whether you choose gels, energy bars, or energy drinks (or maybe even a peanut butter sandwich) – the general recommendation is to consume 1 – 2 ounces (30 – 60 grams) of carbohydrates per hour or 120 to 240 calories per hour during endurance exercise.

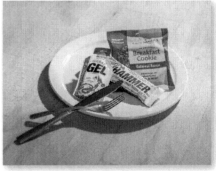

You can't digest large quantities of food while exercising. Your digestive system slows down to provide more blood to your working muscles. If you eat too much, you may get a belly ache or become nauseous.

Fuel After Exercise

First of all, it matters to know WHAT you are recovering from. For the purpose of this book, I am talking about recovery from an extended aerobic effort, such as a two-hour bike ride or long run. You must replenish your muscles' glycogen stores and take care of some muscle repair. I'm not talking about recovery from a hard weight training session where the primary goal is to rebuild muscle.

The general rule of thumb for aerobic recovery is a 3- or 4-to-1 ratio of carbohydrates to protein in your recovery fueling. Whether this is food to chew or drink is up to you.

After you finish exercising, you have a 30-to-60 minute "muscle recovery window." During this time, your body becomes more ready to stock up on stored carbohydrates because the enzyme responsible for glycogen storage *(glycogen synthase)* is elevated instantly after exercise.

Here is the recipe for one of my favorite post-ride smoothies. This smoothie has a 4:1 carbohydrate to protein ratio and about 500 calories. It packs a big recovery punch!

CHOCO-BANANA PB POWER SHAKE (in your blender)
    1 Frozen Banana
    1 TB Peanut Butter (or nut butter of choice)
    1 Scoop Protein powder (vanilla or plain)
    Dark Chocolate Almond Milk to cover
    (Add ice if you like it more milk-shakey)

Hydration, the Color of your Urine, and Muscle Cramps

Hydration: Start every ride with a water bottle (and if you are indoors, include a sweat towel and good ventilation). Hydration is so important I could write an entire book on that alone. For every hour of cycling, you should take in at least 20 ounces of water.

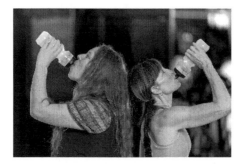

If you exercise for more than an hour, you should take in some electrolytes and carbohydrates for fuel to restock your energy stores as well. Don't chug your water (because that can give you a belly ache). Instead, regularly take small sips or mouthfuls. Don't wait to the end of your ride to drink – take sips throughout.

DRINK A FULL 20 oz. BOTTLE OF WATER EVERY HOUR WHILE YOU RIDE

Then drink another one when you are done. Your muscles depend on good hydration to work efficiently. Think beef jerky (dehydrated) vs. a juicy orange (hydrated). Which do you think is going to be more pliable and give you better function?

Dehydration occurs when the loss of body fluids exceeds the amount taken in. Your body is an amazing self-regulating machine and prefers to keep a balance (homeostasis) of its systems. When dehydration begins, your cells lose fluid, your blood plasma volume falls, and your body has to work harder at basic circulation and function at the cellular level. Your blood pressure may drop. In extreme cases, death can occur.

Don't mess with hydration! Staying hydrated makes everything in your body work better. Think again about this: Do you want your cells to be like beef jerky or like a plump juicy orange?

The Color of Your Urine

Check your hydration by the color and smell of your urine. Darker and smellier urine indicates you may be low on fluids.

- If your urine is a pale yellow like the color of straw with no or little odor = hydrated
- If your urine is honey colored and mild smelling = need fluids
- If your urine is amber colored or with a red or brown tint and strong smelling = need more fluids

    If you feel dehydrated *or have been drinking water but still feel thirsty*, water alone may not do the trick. Your body stays in fluid balance with the help of electrolytes.

What Are Electrolytes Anyway?

Electrolytes are molecules that, when dissolved, have the ability to conduct electricity. Our body functions on a complex balance of positive and negative charges to make things happen such as muscle movement (including cramps), heart beating, and transfer of fluids to cells.

Here is a list of the major electrolytes and common food sources. There are many sports drinks and energy foods offering electrolyte supplementation.

Calcium: Milk, yogurt, cheese, sardines, green leafy vegetables

Potassium: Sweet potatoes, tomatoes, beet greens, bananas, white beans

Magnesium: Spinach and other leafy dark greens, nuts, seeds, fish, beans, peas

Sodium and chloride: Table salt

Phosphate: Found in almost all foods, especially milk, meat, fish

Muscle Cramps

Ever get a muscle cramp while exercising or at night while you sleep? One reason may be you are dehydrated and/or your electrolyte balance is off.

A personal note: I was chronically (mildly) dehydrated for years. I had headaches every morning when I woke up. I was lackluster. After contemplating my nutritional habits, I quit drinking diet sodas and started drinking more water and, magically, my headaches went away. How about that! I keep a bottle of water by my bed, in the car, and on my desk at work, and I always travel with my bike water bottle.

CHAPTER 5

TACKLE YOUR FEARS – MYTHS, MISTAKES, AND YOUR GUIDE TO DON'TS AND DO'S

Yeah, but….maybe you still have some lingering fears about riding a bike. Perhaps the last time you were on one wasn't so fun or was many years ago. I want you to take a whole new approach. You CAN do this and if you take small consistent steps, you WILL see positive changes over time. Cycling, done properly (using the Healthy Knees Secrets to Cycling), will not only help your knees, hips, and ankles, but will also help with managing your weight (cycling can burn oodles of calories) and improving your heart so that everyday tasks are a little easier. BUT FIRST, let's tackle some of your fears.

Myths Debunked
Cycling Myth #1: Riding Inside is Boring

Well, it might be if you hop on a bike without a plan or do something like read a book while you cycle. Yuck. With a good instructor or even our Healthy Knees or Cycle Moles Power to Pedal training videos you always have a purpose for every ride plus motivation and encouragement along the way. Plus, it's addicting (in a good way). It feels GREAT to work hard, get your heart rate up, and breath big. All those endorphins produced by your efforts make you feel good and alive!

For follow-along at home workouts, checkout our Healthy Knees and Cycle Moles videos (as downloads or DVDs) at **www.HealthyKneesBook.com/Videos**

Cycling Myth #2: You Have to Go ALL OUT to get the Most Benefit

No, you don't need to suffer. Training could involve fundamentals, base building, *and* race-type efforts, but the combination of your on-bike activities depends on your goals. You are always in control of how hard you work. Having a coach or program to guide you helps you achieve the appropriate levels of effort.

If you are in a class, no one else really cares what you are doing because they are focused on their own workout. The periodized training we produce in Healthy Knees and Cycle Moles programs plan out your intensity for you so you don't need to worry about working out hard enough. The programs are planned for the appropriate intensity to bring you the most benefit.

When you are just starting out, it is most important to build up strength and stamina and that takes time. Each ride do your best and forget the rest.

Cycling Myth #3: Steady State Workouts Target Fat

I hate this myth! The fitness industry has done a big disservice in touting the whole "fat burning zone" myth.

It is true you burn a larger percentage of fat at lower heart rate. However, interval (high intensity) training burns *more calories overall* and improves your body's ability to burn fat at higher heart rate levels.

Cycling Myth #4: Cycling will Make My Back Hurt

Your back shouldn't hurt when you ride a bike! If it does, your bike is probably set up incorrectly, is the wrong size, the reach to your handle bars is too far, or you have poor body position. All of these things can be fixed and I address them in the "Bike Fit" and "Body Check" sections of this book.

Cycling Myth #5: The Strongest Rider Wins

OK, this is sort of an outdoor thing, but indoor training on technique totally changes this picture. If you take two people with the same strength, the one with the superior technique wins.

Indoor cycling gives you the chance to focus on technique because you are not worrying about road hazards, traffic, or dogs chasing you.

You can focus on a specific aspect of cycling without distraction. And even if you never ride outside, you can be confident you are getting the most out of your indoor experience.

Cycling Myth #6: Only Fit People can Cycle

Peeking into the cycling room can be a little intimidating. I get that. But anyone can ride an indoor cycle because you totally control the intensity and it is easy (no-impact!) on your joints. All you need is a bike: your own bike on a trainer, an indoor cycling bike, or any bike at the gym. Yes, your hiney takes a little time to get used to the saddle (about 2 weeks) but if you follow the "Healthy Knees Secrets to Cycling" you'll feel better, even "down there" (and a pair of padded bike shorts certainly help!).

If you are going to ride outside and haven't done much (or any) before, start small. Even just ride around the block one time. Build from there. I have read countless success stories of individuals who went from zero experience to riding a few miles which grew into much more. There is no distance you must ride, just ride for fun! Ride to lose weight! Ride to make your legs stronger and knees healthier.

Cycling Myth #7: I'm Too Big to Cycle

Cycling is one of the best activities for someone carrying extra pounds because it is easy on your hips, knees, and ankles. Most indoor cycle bikes have a maximum load of 250-350 pounds, and bikes are definitely built to support. If you are concerned about the bike, check with your gym or the bike the manufacturer for the maximum load specifications. You can even ask if the bike seat can be switched for one offering a wider base of support.

Again, start with what you can do. Find a shorter indoor cycling class. Get 10 – 20 minutes on a bike at your club. Find a certified "Healthy Knees" Specialist or Coach. Or put your own bike on a trainer at your home and ride to the "Healthy Knees" indoor cycling videos. Here's the thing, nothing will change to improve your knees until you start taking action with consistency and with persistence. Feeling better does not happen overnight. You can't undo years in just days. Be patient and keep working at it!

You can find these videos at **www.HealthyKneesBook.com/Videos**

Cycling Myth #8: I will Never get Comfortable on that Small Bike Seat

The bike seat, or "saddle," can seem too narrow to ever be comfortable. Good news! If it is your own bike, you can swap out the saddle for a wider, cushier seat for your tush. If you are attending a class, ask if they have a more comfy saddle or a gel seat cover. We offer them at our Club!

That said, it's most important to learn how to sit properly for comfort. Specialists at bike shops can measure the distance between your sit bones to make sure you have the correct saddle width. At first, you may want to have a wider seat for more comfort and some clubs offer that option.

If yours does not, consider purchasing a gel seat cover to give yourself a little more cushion. For comfort, when you are perched on your saddle, do a hip tuck to push your sit bones into the widest part of the seat for the most comfort. Do NOT tip your hips forward. This puts pressure on your pubic bone area.

It may take a couple of weeks for your "hoo-ha" to make peace with the saddle, but pretty soon you won't even notice it.

Cycling Myth #9: I am too Old to Start Cycling

Too old? No way! As long as your doctor says cycling is an appropriate activity for you and you have no other health reasons preventing an aerobic workout, go ahead, get on a bike! If you are not confident in riding outside, indoor training is a great way to start (you can't fall over!).

Work with a Healthy Knees Cycling Specialist or Coach to get a good bike fit and start with all of the healthy parameters I've outlined in this book. I have helped people begin cycling for the first time starting in their 60s, 70s and even into their 80s. Work at your own pace, pay attention to your perceived exertion (how hard you feel you are working), and enjoy the feeling of cycling. You may need to follow the Healthy Knees program for building the strength and balance to stand on your pedals. Success comes with practice and time.

"Cycling has been a wonderful for thing for me. The more I cycled, the better my knees felt" ~ Bob H., retired Ear Nose Throat physician who took up cycling at age 65 and has since competed in local events and the National Masters Road Racing Championships placing 8th in the age 70-74 category.

Cycling Myth #10: I will Do it Wrong or Feel Dumb Because I Don't Know what to Do.

I hope that is why you bought this book: to learn what to expect before you start riding and how to look like a pro even before you get going! Just be sure to follow the advice on how to set up your bike.

If you are in a class, always take a moment to introduce yourself to the instructor and ask them if there is anything you should know before getting started. During class, they can give you the cues on what to do and how to do it. The instructor may ask you a few questions about your level of fitness and if you've ever done indoor cycling because you can never tell just by looking at someone.

Usually other people in cycling classes are pretty helpful because they were in your shoes at some time too. Just say hello and ask questions if you don't know.

Common Mistakes
Pedaling Speed and Tension: Too Slow/Too Much and Too Fast/Too Little

Most people start out pedaling very slowly with too much tension. Each pedal stroke is a grind and cycling becomes painful. High resistance and slow pedal speed puts more torque force in your knee joint for every pedal stroke.

Conversely, in some indoor cycling classes I've seen people pedaling wildly at 130 RPM. Elite racers have the muscle control and strength to do this; most of the rest of us are putting our knees at risk. Almost all spinning style bikes have a weighted fly-wheel to help with pedal momentum. When you get pedaling that fast, it is likely there is very little resistance (so you CAN pedal fast) and the fly-wheel is pushing you rather than you controlling your speed. This puts your knees at risk! One wrong move and TWINK! Ouch goes the knees.

In Cycle Moles and Healthy Knees Cycling, we teach you the appropriate parameters of how fast to pedal and how much tension to add to give you optimal control. If you want to pedal fast, it is far better to pedal at 100 to 110 RPM and add tension to make it a challenge. You build stronger muscles and better control.

Only Pushing Down or "Pedaling Bricks"

When you learned how to ride a bike that is exactly what you were taught: push down on the pedals. In fact, if you don't have your feet attached somehow (toe cages or bike shoes with cleats), that *is* all you can do. This is a quadriceps-dominant way to pedal and there are more opportunities to engage more of your leg muscle to improve your pedaling efficiency, create more power, and strengthen your knees.

Remember the round pedal stroke! Push down, pull back (like you are scraping mud off the bottom of your shoes), lift up, and kick over the top. This movement doesn't come naturally for most people, so we practice this in our sessions. Even the Pros need to practice their pedal stroke. (More on this technique in "Healthy Knees Secrets to Cycling".)

Moving your Upper Body

New cyclists often rock their upper body side to side with each pedal stroke. This shows me they are only pushing down on the pedals (instead of using a complete pedal stroke) and may have a weak core. Always try to keep your upper body quiet, thinking about making the work happen from your hips down.

Tension in your Shoulders

I have to remind myself to pull my shoulders out of my ears! As you get tired or the intensity increases, you may find you start holding more tension in your shoulders and they start shrugging up toward your ears.

Try this with me now: shrug and hold your shoulders up toward your ears, take in a deep breath, and blow out releasing all of the tension in your shoulders. This relaxed state is where you want to be. If you find you get tense while you ride (indoors or out), try this inhale-and-release technique.

Dont's and Do's

Don'ts

Don't wear Earphones on the Road

Your ability to hear activity around you while you are cycling keeps you safe. Dogs barking? Cars coming? Train on the tracks? Besides, there are so many relaxing sounds when you ride – children laughing, hidden waterfalls, and birds singing – why would you want to miss that?

Don't Lift Weights on Bike

Why not? When lifting weights or stretching on a bike, proper body position is compromised and your back and knees are placed at risk. The weights you are lifting are usually significantly less than what you can do with your feet planted on the floor.

If you want to lift weights, please get off the bike and pursue it with proper body alignment.

If You Wouldn't Do It Outside, Don't Do It Inside

I hold this credo: never do anything on a bike *indoors* you wouldn't do while riding your bike outside.

Silly moves like pushups, rapid up and down moves, and weird arm waving don't get you in better shape and may injure you. Even stretching on a bike, while pedaling, may tweak something. If you want to do strength training or stretching, get off the bike, put your body in the proper position, and get the most benefit from it.

Do's (The 3 Hs)

Helmet

This is worth repeating: when riding outside, always, always wear your helmet. It doesn't take any speed to fall and have a head injury. Mussed hair is worth saving your head. Traumatic brain injuries are serious.

Hydrate

Hydration has already been mentioned, but it is so important it is also worth bringing up again. Drink a 20-ounce bottle of water for every hour you cycle. Drink another bottle of water after you ride. Your body recovers more quickly and you'll feel much better.

Have Fun

Cycling, whether indoor, outside, or both, can be a joyous part of your day. You can ride for fitness, competition, to lose weight, commuting, sightseeing, adventure travel, or simply because it is fun!

I hope now you feel more prepared for getting on a bike. You've chosen your bike, you'll ride inside or outside (or maybe both), you know what to wear and how to fuel your body. Congratulations! You are ready. It is time. And OH BOY are we going to have fun!

Cycling is always the best part of my day. Here is the way I see it: I never look at riding my bike as a chore because the time on my bike is all about me. I think it is the most valuable part of my day since I am doing something good for my knees and my health. Taking care of yourself is not a selfish thing...it is actually self-less. If you are as healthy as you can be, you can become the best you. The best you is able to take care of all the people you love and the work you care about better than any other version of you. The "best you" helps you give better to others. If you are ready to become a healthier, better you, (with stronger knees!) let me share the four Healthy Knees Secrets with you.

CHAPTER 6

HEALTHY KNEES SECRETS TO CYCLING: THE 4 HEALTHY KNEES FOUNDATIONS

Doctors often recommend cycling for rehabilitation from a knee injury or to strengthen aching knees. But they don't tell you *how* to cycle, because that is not their specialty. That is why I am here! The "how" makes all the difference. You can make your knees *worse* if you do not have your bike set up correctly, if you pedal too slowly with too much force, or if you go too fast without enough tension. You can be terribly uncomfortable if you don't know the proper body position.

When I walk through the workout area of our gym, I see the "wrong" way on a bike all of the time. Of course I stop and make suggestions because the Four Healthy Knees Foundations are not intuitive. They are learned and you need to practice. I've been riding for years and I still practice these elements every time I ride. It always starts with proper *bike* set up which sets *you* up for success. Proper body position (especially your hips, elbows, and wrists) make you much more comfortable on your bike. If you get fatigued while you ride, you may find your elbows going straight, your shoulders scrunched up by your ears, and your back arched…just remind yourself "Body Check!" and relax.

Yes, there *are* right and wrong ways to cycle. I am sharing my secrets to help you skip the wrong and go straight to the optimal set up for your bike, your body, and your knees. It took me years and thousands of miles to figure this out. I want you to have this information now so you get on a *healthier path right away*. Without further ado, here they are, the four Healthy Knees Foundations for making cycling great for your knees. Let's get started.

HK Foundation #1: The 5 Secrets to Bike Fit (Do This First!)

Cycling is a repetitive motion activity and if you are pedaling at 90 rotations per minute for 30 minutes that's 2700 rotations pedaled for each knee! This is why it is crucial to have your bike set up optimally for your body and according to the geometry of the bike

You can use these tips for any upright stationary bike. If you are attending an indoor class, arrive early and introduce yourself to the instructor. He or she may help you set up your bike. But since I want you to be prepared, I'll tell you how to do this on your own (so everyone else looks at you in awe).

You want to be comfortable on your bike, right? The Healthy Knees "Bike Fit and Comfort Tips" video explains this (**www.HealthyKneesBook.com/bonus**), but here it is written down for your reference. If you must reset a bike each time you hop on, write down your settings so you don't need to measure every time.

For the purpose of pedal position, we'll use a clock.

12 o'clock is your foot at the top of the pedal circle,

3 o'clock is your forward foot pushing down, (half-way to the bottom)

6 o'clock is your foot at the bottom of the pedal circle,

9 o'clock is your back foot pulling up on your pedals, (half-way up)

When your feet are at 3 o'clock and 9 o'clock, they are parallel with the ground.

Bike Fit #1: Foot Position

Place the widest part of your shoe on the pedal, not your arch, not your heel. Toe cages are designed to accommodate a variety of lengths of feet. If you have a smaller shoe size, you probably won't need to push your toe all the way to the end of the toe cage. That would not be good foot position. When pedaling, the ball of your foot should be centered on the pedal.

Bike Fit #2: Seat Height (Knee Extension)

For an upright stationary bike, start by finding your hip bone and poke it with your thumb. Then, hold your hand out flat next to the seat, as shown. That is the first guess for seat height.

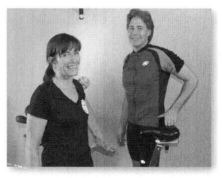

If you are on an outdoor bike, you'll need to balance in a stationary position (put your bike on a trainer or hold yourself upright against a counter) and have a friend look at your leg angle.

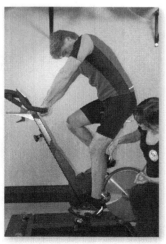

Seated on the bike, pedal for about 20 rotations the come to a stop with one leg at full extension (this should be at about "5 o'clock" for pedal position). It's good if you have a mirror or a friend to help you get in the correct position.

With the ball of your foot on the pedal, your knee should have a 25- to 35-degree bend. This is a slight bend.

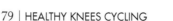

If you don't happen to have a goniometer, a smartphone app, or other tool to measure your angle of bend, try this:

While holding your lower pedal at 5 o'clock, move your heel to the front of the pedal. Your leg should be straight. (See picture.)

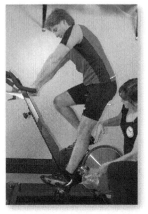

- When your heel is at the front of the pedal, if you still have a bend in your knee, your saddle height is probably too low. If you are too low, you are missing out on power you can put into your pedals.
- If you can't reach the front of the pedal with your heel or need to shift your hips to reach it, your saddle height is probably too high. If you are too high you may experience pain in the back of your knee (hyperextension) or in your low back because you rock your hips to get power into your pedals.

Bike Fit #3: Knee Over Pedal

It should be possible to adjust the position of your saddle closer to or farther away from the handlebars. The most important part of location of your saddle fore/aft is its relationship to the bottom bracket (where the pedal arms connect to the bike). On your body, we measure the position of your knee to your pedal.

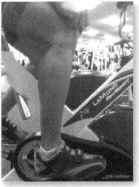

While on your bike, bring your feet to the same level and parallel with the floor. On a clock, this would be the 3 o'clock and 9 o'clock position.

Check your position: When you are in the cycling position (hands on handle bars) and looking down at your forward foot in the 3 o'clock position, you should be able to see the front part of your foot from the widest part of your foot (just behind your toes) to your toe of your shoe. If you hung a plumb bob (or a weighted string) from the bony knob on your shin just below your knee (tibial tuberosity) front of your knee, it should line up with the ball of your foot and where the pedal connects to the pedal arm, plus or minus ¾ inch (about 2 centimeters).

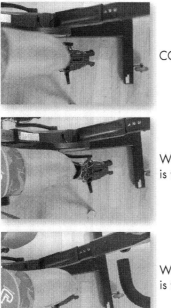

CORRECT, can see ball of foot to toes

WRONG, can see whole foot means saddle is too far back

WRONG, can't see foot means saddle is too far foreward

- If you see *more* of your foot, move your saddle toward your handlebars.
- If you see *less* of your foot, move your saddle away from your handlebars.

- When pedaling, if you feel pain in the front of your knee, you may be out of alignment. This often means your saddle is too close to your handlebars and your knee – at the 3 o'clock position – is past the mid-point of the pedal. This puts too much force in the knee joint and can cause discomfort. To fix this, move your saddle back (away from the handlebars) and check your foot position at the 3 o'clock.

Bike Fit #4: Handlebar Height

On an indoor bike, there really is no need to "get aero" (tuck down against your bike frame so you are pushing less wind) since you are stationary and not pushing through the air. Comfort is the rule. In general, you want to choose a comfortable handlebar height. Look for a body angle of 20 degrees to 45-degree lean forward from your hips. You should feel 40% of your body weight in your hands and 60% in your butt on the saddle[13].

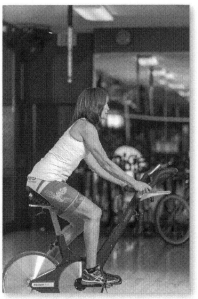

CORRECT body angle

Bike Fit #5: Handlebar Fore/Aft

In general, you want a 90-degree angle from your torso to your arms. Stretching out farther than 90 degrees may cause upper body discomfort. You may have to monkey with your handlebar height and fore/aft adjustments to get this setting correct. Again, it is helpful to have a mirror or a friend to check your position. Remember you want a weight distribution of 40% in your hands and 60% on your saddle.

---

13 Serotta International Cycling Institute, *Personalized Class Companion Manual*, (2013) page 40.

YOUR BIKE FIT CHECKLIST

____ Foot Position (Widest part of foot or ball of foot on pedal)

____ Seat Height (At full extension of leg and pedal position at "5 o'clock" 25-35° bend in knee while foot is level to ground)

____ Knee Over Pedal (Seat Fore/Aft) (With feet parallel to ground, drop a plumb bob from the tibial tuberosity below your knee which should point at the center of the pedal or +/- ¾ inch or 2 centimeters.)

____ Handlebar Height (Back angle at 20 – 45°. Weight distribution 40% in hands, 60% in saddle.)

____ Handle Bar Fore/Aft (Torso to arm angle is 90°. Weight distribution 40% in hands, 60% in saddle.)

Download the Bike Fit and Comfort Tips Checklist at
www.HealthyKneesBook.com/Resources.

HK Foundation #2: The 6 Body Checks and Comfort Tips

After your bike is adjusted (see "Bike Fit," above), it is time to get comfortable on it! When you are riding along and some part of you becomes uncomfortable, think "Body Check!" Mentally check your six points of alignment and make an adjustment.

Body Check #1: Foot Position

Remember your foot alignment: the widest part of your foot should be on the pedal next to where the pedal connects to the pedal arm. In general, your foot should be parallel to the bike frame with your toes and heels in alignment. Your knee issues may come into play, here. It may be more comfortable for you to have a heel or toe pointing in.

The best way to figure out your optimal foot position: have a proper bike set up and put your shoe on the pedal in the proper position. Pedal a few strokes to let your body fall into its natural alignment (do not clip in or tighten your foot in a toe cage). Now, have someone else look at your foot position and notice if your heel or toe is rotated closer to the bike frame or is parallel to the frame.

Understanding your body's natural position helps you with comfort. This information is critical if you wear bike shoes with cleats, because you must adjust your shoe cleat to give your foot the desired position on your pedal. Be sure to read the section on bike shoes and pedals for more information about pedal types. This is important for your knee and hip comfort.

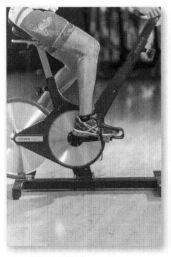

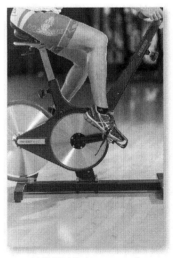

CORRECT foot position
0 – 25 degrees

WRONG (tippy toes)
foot position

Many people start out with "tippy toes" on the bike, meaning the toes are pointed down and heels are raised like they are walking on their toes. Unfortunately, this tippy toe position sends a lot of your pedaling force out through your toes instead of down into the pedal. Rather than tippy toe, keep your foot flat. Feel a push from the ball of your foot through to the pedal. Lower your heel to a 0 to 25-degree angle from parallel with the floor throughout your pedal stroke.

If you are an advanced-level cyclist, you'll know there are a number of pedaling techniques including "ankleing" or flexing and extending your ankle for more power. If you know about these and practice them, by all means continue. For the beginner, however, I have found the foot position providing the biggest power benefit is a more flat position throughout the pedal stroke.

Body Check #2: Knee Position (tucked in, parallel, flared out)

Ideally, for recreational cyclists, when you sit on the saddle and have your feet in the proper position on a bike, both knees should point straight ahead. "Ideally" is the operative word here. If you have knee issues, there may be other factors at play.

Your knee problems and body mechanics determine, to a large part, what direction your knees want to go. *If it does not cause pain*, you'll want to point them both straight forward in alignment with your lower leg.

Your knee position depends on three connecting joints of your leg: ankle, knee, and hip. If some body part is out of alignment, it affects your entire kinetic chain from your foot to your knee to your hip and on up to your lower back. Notice your body position and try some adjustments. Hopefully this alleviates discomfort. If it causes more pain, don't do it!

Knee issues

Your knee condition dictates if your knee is tucked in toward the bike frame, parallel to it, or flared out. The preferred position is parallel or tucked in (you'll see the pros do this, making themselves more aerodynamic.)

Foot position

Your foot position may be dictated in part by your knee and your hip. If your heel is rotated "IN," your knee is probably pointing out. If your heel is pointing "OUT," your knee is pointing in. Place the ball of your foot on the pedal even if you are "heel in" or "heel out".

Hip position

Hips should be neutral with your sit bones on the widest part of the seat. You do not want your back hunched (likely a posterior pelvic tilt) or sunken (an anterior tilt to your pelvis). Mostly, you want to feel the pressure of the saddle on your sit bones, not on your pubic bone area (that is not comfortable for anyone!).

Years ago, I had been experiencing lower back pain for a long time and finally went in for a professional bike fit. Sometimes it is best to have someone else evaluate your form on a bike. The expert noticed I was lifting my left heel and my left hip was rotated back. I did not realize I was doing this! Without looking at yourself in a mirror, it is hard to see such things. I was unconsciously making this adjustment to protect my left knee (the worse of the two) by reducing the angle of the knee bend at the top of the pedal stroke (since I had scooted my left hip back on the saddle). To re-learn proper alignment, I spent an entire winter on trainer rides in my basement working on dropping that heel and rotating my hips correctly. My lower back pain went away! I still find, when I get tired on a ride, I tend to return to this poor position and must continually do my "body check."

Body Check #3: Sit Bones on the Saddle

Here is a tip to make things more comfortable "down there" from the get-go: Do not tip forward with your hips (which puts painful pressure on your pubic bone area and the -ahem- soft tissues down there); instead, push your sit bones into the back of the saddle (where there is the most padding on your hiney and your saddle), keep your hips square, and bend forward at the waist. If you've ever taken Pilates, this is like doing a slight "C-Curl" into the saddle.

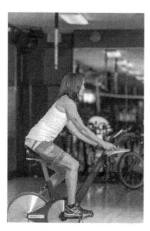

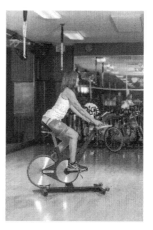

CORRECT back position
with neutral spine

WRONG (sway)
back position with
anterior pelvic tilt.

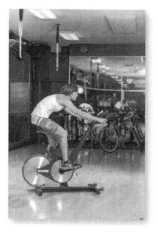

WRONG (hunched)
back position with
posterior pelvic tilt

Body Check #4: Flat Back and Relaxed Shoulders

Keep your back flat as you lean toward your handlebars. Your core comes in to play here, supporting your upper torso and giving you stability. A strong core helps keep your back happy and reduce aches and pains.

Check yourself - is your back arched or hunched when you ride? Try flattening it out for prolonged comfort.

Pull your shoulders out of your ears! Right now, take a deep breath inhale and squeeze your shoulders up to your ears; as you exhale drop your shoulders and completely let out all of the tension. This is your ideal position.

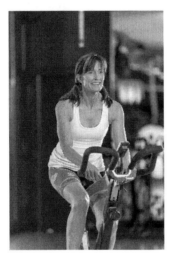 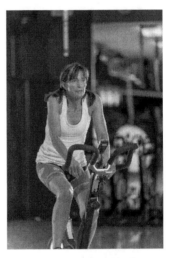

CORRECT relaxed shoulders   WRONG scrunched, tense shoulders

Body Check #5: Al Dente Elbows

Think pasta (which is what you've earned after your bike rides – oh, don't get distracted!). Your elbows should not be uncooked (stiff) or overcooked (too bent) but instead should be "al dente" with a slight bend. A soft elbow with about 15 to 25 degrees of bend reminds you to keep light tension with your hands on the handlebars. If you have a death grip or lean heavily on your bars, you are putting a lot of tension into your hands, wrists, and shoulders. This causes fatigue, and it is something I see when people get tired or are inexperienced. It also may be a sign of a weak core! Instead of stiff arms, use your core to hold you up.

A slight bend in your elbows helps with circulation. Your hands and shoulders stay fresh. If your hands go numb when you ride, your wrists may be cocked, your arms might be stiff and straight, or you put too much weight on the handlebars (which may call for a handlebar adjustment).

A slight bend in your elbows when you ride outdoors also acts as a shock absorber. If your arms are stick straight, you are transmitting all of the vibration from the road right through to your shoulders and up your neck.

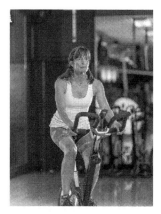

CORRECT soft bend
(al dente) in elbow

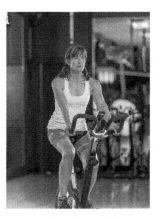

WRONG Stiff
(uncooked pasta!) elbows

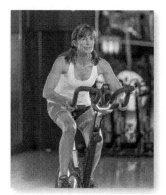

WRONG too much bend
(overcooked pasta) elbows

Body Check #6: Rolled Wrists

Take a look at your wrists when you hold the handlebars in the various positions. You want a continuous long line from your forearm to the top of your hand instead of a bent or "cocked" wrist. This is key for circulation in your hands. Also, if your hands go numb, you may be gripping the handlebars too tightly. The median nerve runs from your forearm to the palm of your hand to innervate your thumb and fingers (except your pinky). This nerve runs through a narrow rigid passageway of ligament and bones between the wrist and palm of your hand (called the carpal tunnel). If you hold your wrist in a bent position while pressing weight on it, you put a significant amount of pressure on that small opening. This can numb your hands. If your pinky finger goes numb, it may be from putting too much pressure on the outside of your hand. Straighten thy wrists!

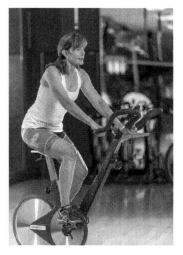 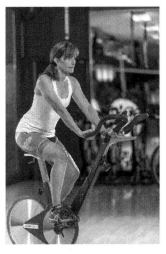

CORRECT long line forearm to wrist

WRONG cocked wrists

YOUR BODY CHECK CHECKLIST

_____ Foot Position (0 – 25° lift of heel)

_____ Knee Position (Knee in line with foot, not flared out)

_____ Hips (Sit Bones on Saddle, not pubic bone)

_____ Flat Back and Relaxed Shoulders

_____ "Al Dente" Elbows (soft bend)

_____ Rolled Wrists (not cocked!)

Download the Bike Fit and Comfort Tips Checklist at
www.HealthyKneesBook.com/Resources.

HK Foundation #3: 4 Secrets to Pedal Stroke Zones (Are you Pedaling Bricks or Circles?)

Did you know there is more to pedaling a bike (and knee happiness) than just pushing down on the pedals? When pedaling a bike, the power phase is from 30° to 150° (or 1:00 to 5:00 on a clock). It is initiated from your gluteus muscles and continued by your quadriceps.

When you have your feet attached to the pedal by toe cage or clipless pedals, you have the ability to engage more muscles and support your knees better. The four parts to the pedal stroke are Downstroke, Bottomstroke, Upstroke, and Topstroke.

To help visualize the circle pedal stroke, use zones on a clock. 12:00 o'clock is at the top of the circle (in the Topstroke), 3:00 o'clock is foot forward half-way down (in the Downstroke), 6:00 is the lowest pedal point and is in the Bottomstroke, and 9:00 o'clock is halfway up on the backside of your pedal stroke while you lift up in the Upstroke.

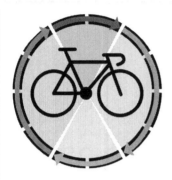

Pedal Stroke Zones

There are many debates about the effectiveness of using the parts of the pedal stroke for elite athletes (do you lift up or not in the upstroke?). However, for good knee health, let's all learn to pedal more efficiently and actively engage more muscles throughout the pedal stroke. This means it is NOT all about just pushing down.

"Pedaling Bricks" is a term used to describe the "thud" or a dead spot at the bottom of your pedal stroke and even a "thud" at the top. This occurs when you are mostly just pushing down on the pedals. Instead, let's turn those bricks into circles!

Downstroke

This is what you learned as a kid. Just push down on the pedals. It is the most powerful part of your pedal stroke, using predominantly your gluteus (hip extensors) and quadriceps (lower leg extensor) muscles.

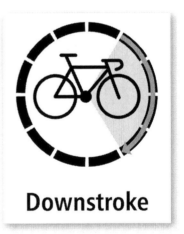

Downstroke

What to Feel: Pressure on the ball of your foot as you push against the pedal

Where on the Clock: 1:00 o'clock to 5:00 o'clock.

Bottomstroke

Pull your foot back like you are wiping mud off the bottom of your shoe or you are a bull about to charge. Muscles recruited include your calf (ankle plantar flexor), front of shin (ankle dorsiflexor), and knee flexors (hamstrings).

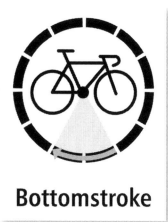

Bottomstroke

What to Feel: Your heel against the back of your shoe as you pull your foot back.

Where on the Clock: 5:00 to 7:00 o'clock

Upstroke

Lift up like you have puppet strings attached to your knees and are using your whole thigh to lift up your leg. Muscles recruited include hamstrings (knee flexors) and iliopsoas muscle group (hip flexors) and tensor fascia latae (hip abduction).

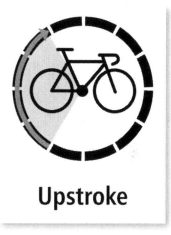

Upstroke

What to Feel: As you lift, keep your foot in a 0 - 25 degree position from the ground, feel the top of your foot against the top of your shoe as you lift. Think about keeping your heel down - do not pull up with your heel, pull up with the *top* of your foot.

Where on the Clock: 7:00 to 11:00 o'clock

Topstroke

Kick over the top of the pedal stroke as if you are kicking a ball with the toe of your foot. Engage your quadriceps muscles (knee extensors) and gluteus (hip extensors) muscles.

What to Feel: Like you are shooting your foot forward. You may notice your RPM just increased because you've become a little more efficient.

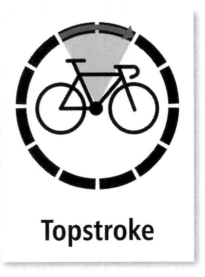

Topstroke

Where on the Clock: 11:00 to 1:00 o'clock

HK Foundation #4: Pedal Speed and Tension (The Healthy Knees Rules)

Most people start out pedaling relatively slowly both indoors and outside. Slow pedaling requires you to use higher tension or a harder gear and this slow pedal speed puts more torque force in your knee joint on every push of the pedals. One of the things we teach is a better pedal speed with the right amount of tension. This engages more muscles and reduces the joint force on each pedal stroke. We coach you in this method in our cycling classes and videos.

On the other hand, spinning as fast as you can with little tension is not good either. Indoor cycling bikes usually have a weighted flywheel that, once it gets going, can carry your feet if you are not in control. This puts your knees at risk! If you find you are pedaling along and your hips start bumping in the saddle, this shows you are not in control of the pedals and they are controlling you! To correct for this, either slow your pedal speed or add more tension. You'll stop hopping around and regain control.

Healthy Knee Pedal Speed Rule: 60-110 RPM

In general, we recommend you keep your pedal speed (indoors) between 60 RPM and 110 RPM. If you start going slower than 60 RPM, take off some tension and save your knees. If you are pedaling faster than 110 RPM, add tension, build muscle control, and earn that speed!

The base range I like to see for most cyclists is 85-95 RPM (don't worry if you can't do this now: if you follow the Healthy Knees workouts you'll get there sooner than you think!). Once you build the muscle control to do this, your knees feel better. You'll find you can ride longer with less fatigue. Practice pedaling with tension at all of the pedal speeds in the Healthy Knees range. This helps build more strength and expands neuro-muscular control.

That said, there will be times you pedal slower than 60 RPM (for example, when you are on a hill). We teach hill climbing techniques in our videos and live classes, and can help you become stronger and faster while saving your knees.

If you must drop below 60 RPM, I recommend standing to do so. It changes the angle of your leg and you have your body weight working with you to help push through the resistance. Yes, you do more work and it is harder to stand and pedal; you've shifted your primary weight bearing from your behind on your saddle to your feet on your pedals. While standing, keep your knees soft, your weight in your feet (not on your handlebars), and your hips over your pedals.

> *If you don't have a cadence meter on your bike,*
> *how do you know how fast you are pedaling?*
>
> *Pedal for a 15-second count, tap one knee at the top of each pedal stroke. Multiply this count by 4 for your RPM (rotations per minute)*
>
> 15 Second Count:
> 15 Taps = 60 RPM
> 18 Taps = 72 RPM
> 20 Taps = 80 RPM
> 23 Taps = 92 RPM
> 25 Taps = 100 RPM
> 27 Taps = 108 RPM
>
> Check out the video at **www.HealthyKneesBook.com/Resources** to see exactly how to count out your RPM.

Learning the Healthy Knees Secrets to Cycling for *how* to pedal gives you more power to your pedals and, by recruiting more muscles in your legs, makes you stronger (and your effort easier). You become more efficient. Practicing how fast and how hard to pedal is a gauge for your knees: as you get stronger, you can add more tension and keep your knees happy at the same time. At first, you don't want to pile on the tension because you haven't built the knee stability and muscle strength to support it. Too much tension may make your knees sore. How *do* you gauge how much tension to add? We explore "how hard is hard for you" in the next chapter.

CHAPTER 7

HOW HARD SHOULD YOU WORK?

How hard is "hard" for you? It is subjective and it is a learned perception. In our Healthy Knees and Cycle Moles classes, we talk about the work level all of the time. If you are sitting on a bike throwing a leg around a pedal every so often while reading a magazine… is that hard? Unlikely. Are you doing yourself any good? Not so much. To get benefit from your exercise, you must put some effort into it. Your perception of what is hard has a lot to do with your experience in exercise. If you are (or were) a competitive athlete, your expectation of "hard" is different from someone who is new to exercise. The good news is: as you put more effort into your exercise you get stronger, you improve your confidence of what you can achieve, and you raise the level of what is "hard" for you. Gains in strength and ability happen in just a couple of weeks if you follow the Healthy Knees plan.

It is OK to get your heart rate up and I want you to start making a relationship between how hard you think you are working and what your heart is actually doing. Your heart rate, recovery, and resting beats per minute (bpm) tell a story about your heart health. Not only is cycling wonderful for your knees (and hips and ankles), it is great for your heart. Double Bonus!

Building up movement to a moderate or vigorous level has numerous benefits to your cardiovascular system. These positive changes begin to occur in just a few weeks!

- Heart pumps more blood per beat (becomes more efficient!)
- You can exercise at higher intensity (higher heart rates) without feeling fatigued
- Your volume of oxygen breathed in and out expands
- Your body better uses the oxygen in your bloodstream
- Your heart recovery rate improves (going from high heart rate to lower recovery heart rate quicker)
- Your resting heart rate lowers. (This is good! It means your heart is more efficient.)

If you are not used to intensive exercise, start gradually with a 10- to 15-minute session. Increase the amount of time you exercise as you get stronger.

You are in Control

One of the fears I hear about indoor cycling is, "I could never work that hard." You are always in control and really, the other people in the class do not care what you are doing (except the instructor). The beauty of a stationary bike is everyone starts and ends in the same place!

- If you are on a spinning-style bike, there is a tension knob or lever you move to adjust how hard (resistance or tension) it is to pedal.
- If you are on a club bike, you can use a program to automatically adjust your tension (you have the ability to increase or decrease resistance at every interval), or you can switch to manual and adjust it yourself.
- If you are on your own bike mounted to a trainer, you shift gears to make it harder or easier to pedal.

RPE: Rate of Perceived Exertion

How hard do you feel you are working (RPE)? There are a number of different rating scales you can use. I've developed a simple one that also correlates to heart rate training zones.

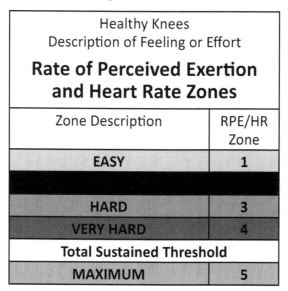

Healthy Knees Description of Feeling or Effort **Rate of Perceived Exertion and Heart Rate Zones**	
Zone Description	RPE/HR Zone
EASY	1
HARD	3
VERY HARD	4
Total Sustained Threshold	
MAXIMUM	5

Zone 1   Easy

This is your warm up, recovery pace, and cool down. In this zone, you are preparing your body for activity or returning to rest. You can carry on a conversation easily.

Zone 2   Moderate

You feel like you are doing just a bit of work in this zone and you could sustain it for a long time. While still a relatively low level of effort, this zone has significant health benefits and works to make your aerobic engine (using fat for fuel) more efficient. You can carry on a conversation comfortably.

Zone 3   Hard

In this zone you know you are working hard and your breathing shifts in frequency as your intensity increases. You improve your functional cardiovascular system. There is increased blood flow to your muscles. Working in this zone helps the heart increase in strength so you can exercise longer before becoming fatigued. Talking is limited to shorter sentences.

Zone 4   Very hard

This zone is reached by going harder and may push you out of your comfort zone. Here you get faster and fitter, increasing your heart rate as you transition from aerobic to anaerobic training at the top of Zone 4. This is where you notice changes in breathing patterns to faster, heavy, and hard. Trained athletes can stay in this zone for long periods, but for some people training every day in Z4 may lead to overtraining. Talking is limited to a few words.

TOTAL SUSTAINED THRESHOLD (see below)

Zone 5   Maximum effort

This is the equivalent of working "all out" and is used mostly as an interval training regimen. Exertion at this level can only be done in short time amounts. You definitely feel like you are making a maximum effort and your breathing accelerates to panting. Even world-class athletes can stay in this zone for only a few minutes at a time. It is not a zone most people select for exercise since working in this zone is uncomfortable. You are working too hard to talk at all except form maybe a word or two.

Total Sustained Threshold (TST)

Let's talk about the threshold. There are many ways to measure your body's metabolic response to exercise. The anaerobic threshold is commonly measured by blood lactate (lactate threshold) or ventilator gases (ventilatory threshold). Much research has been done on both methods and they occur close to the same time.

For the purpose of our discussion, consider the threshold to be the point at which an athlete can sustain the highest workload without a significant change in breathing pattern, from strong and steady changing to panting or gasping. The threshold represents the point at which the body's aerobic engine is working as hard as it can to convert fat (adipose tissue) to energy. When you need *more* energy because you want to go faster or harder, you need a supplemental fuel source. Enter your turbo booster glycogen (stored carbohydrates)! Glycogen is kind of like a dirty fuel. When your body converts fat to energy there is no "by-product." But when your body converts glycogen to energy, you get an "exhaust" of carbon dioxide (CO_2). As you generate more CO_2, you breathe harder to blow it out of your system. Ah ha! That is why you start panting. Your body seeks to rid itself of the CO_2, replacing it with oxygen.

This really is a very complex process and at no time are you using *only* fat or *only* carbohydrates to create energy. Your body is amazing at using the systems it needs to get the job done.

Once you cross your personal threshold, are panting, working "all out," you've entered Zone 5. You cannot sustain that work level for more than 30 seconds. You are also using up your precious (and limited) stores of glycogen. A note: Some elite athletes have trained their bodies to withstand greater amounts of lactic acid and have developed a high "pain tolerance" to function at this level.

What is "Bonking" or "Hitting the Wall"?

The feeling of Bonking or Hitting the Wall is a sudden sensation you are out of energy. Your arms and legs feel like lead, you get dizzy, you may even hallucinate. You are forced to stop moving.

Biologically, you have just experienced complete glycogen depletion (remember, glycogen is the stored form of carbohydrates found in your muscles and liver.) Without this fuel source, you cannot create the energy your muscles need to keep functioning at a high level. It is imperative you eat something with simple carbohydrates as soon as you can.

Bonks can usually be avoided by eating a diet with adequate carbohydrates (portions vary depending on if you are an endurance athlete, weekend warrior, or couch potato). If you are exercising vigorously for more than an hour, consume carbohydrates through drinks or easily-digestible foods. Help your body recover faster after a long bout of exercise by replenishing glycogen stores within an hour of completing your exercise.

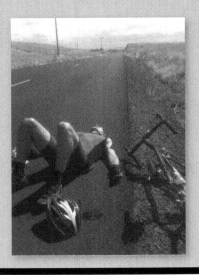

I developed the idea of Total Sustained Threshold (TST) as I was evaluating the factors that go into the highest level of intensity an individual can sustain. "Sustain" is the key word; once you surpass your TST heart rate, you cannot maintain that workload for long. The key is to develop your ability to sustain work just below your threshold at your maximum sustainable heart rate and power.

Now here is the important part: It is not just your physical ability, but also your mental toughness that determines your TST.

"You are stronger than you think you are;
you can do more than you think you can."[14]

Make this your mantra.

For example, if you are new to interval training, you may not be used to pushing yourself to those upper limits. Heck, you might not even know what those limits are in terms of heart rate or how you are supposed to feel when you perform at that level.

But a seasoned athlete who knows their heart rate training zones can work at each level and build the mental tenacity to stick with it... even when it gets uncomfortable and there is a certain amount of physical discomfort. In Healthy Knees and Cycle Moles training, we help you understand each zone of effort and build the stamina and mental toughness to sustain the work.

TST = PHYSICAL ABILITY + MENTAL TOUGHNESS

You can see this in trained athletes who have the ability to keep their mental focus even when their bodies are tired. As you train at this level, you develop the ability to stay mentally tougher for longer. So, let's talk about how you feel and what your heart is up to.

---

14 I've modified this saying from the original "You are better than you think you are, you can do more than you think you can" *from Ken Chlouber, founder of the 100 mile Leadville race series.*

Heart Rate Training

There are many ways to measure your heart's response to activity. The function of your cardiovascular system is to move blood throughout your body, transporting nutrients, respiratory gasses, and other materials.

Everyone's heart rate is unique and is determined by a variety of factors including:

- Genetics
- Age
- Exercise
- Health (fever, illness)
- Medicines
- Heart conditions
- Sleep quantity and quality

Here is important information about heart rate response to exercise:

Heart Rate Follows Effort

Generally, your heart rate lags behind physical effort by 30 to 60 seconds depending on how hard you are working. Understanding the correlation between how hard you *think* you are working and your heart's *actual* response is key to gauging your intensity.

If you know your heart rate zones, you can adjust your level of intensity according to your heart rate readings. Sometimes you'll need to work harder and sometimes you'll need to back off.

If you don't know your heart rate training zones, start to notice how you feel (RPE Zones 1-5) and your associated heart rates. Write it down. With consistent cardio exercise (2 or 3 times per week), record it each time; in a few weeks see if there is any difference.

Recovery After an Intense Interval

Your heart's recovery rate communicates important information about your heart health.

Only perform exercise that is approved by your doctor

To determine your one-minute recovery rate immediately after a peak intensity effort (vigorous activity), count your heart rate in beats per minute. Recover from your effort with low intensity activity or rest. Count your heart rate again one minute later.

If you aren't wearing a heart rate monitor, count your heart rate for 15 seconds by pressing your index finger on your pulse either at your wrist or carotid artery in your neck. Multiply the number by four to get your beats per minute.

Now, subtract your one-minute rate from your peak exercise rate:

Peak exercise bpm _____ - 1 min. heart rate bpm _____ = Recovery Heart Rate _____

According to the Heart Zones ™ manual, your Recovery Heart Rate is evaluated for fitness:

Fewer 10 beats = extreme caution

11-20 beats = low

21-40 beats = good

41-50 beats = excellent

More than 50 beats = fit athlete

It is a good idea to consult a doctor if your Recovery Heart rate is 10 or fewer beats per minute.

Resting Heart Rate

The lower your heart rate at rest, the better your heart is working as a pump.

According to the Mayo Clinic, a normal resting heart rate for adults ranges from 60 to 100 beats per minute. In general, a lower resting heart rate suggests more efficient heart function and better cardiovascular fitness. A fit athlete may have a resting heart rate in the 40-60 bpm range.

Resting heart rate is influenced by many factors:

- Physical fitness
- Medications
- Body size and weight
- Emotions
- Body position
- Environmental conditions (air temperature, wind)
- Hydration
- Sleep quality and quantity

How to measure your resting heart rate:

First thing in the morning, while you are lying in bed (after the shock of the alarm has worn off), use your index finger to take a 15-second count of your pulse at your wrist or carotid artery in your neck. Multiplying this number by four gives your heart rate beats per minute. Record your resting heart rate daily for one week so you have a baseline from which to measure yourself.

A change in resting heart rate can indicate different things.

- An *increase* in resting heart rate may show you are fighting a cold or illness, you are overtraining, you are decreasing in physical fitness, or you may have a cardiac condition (see your doctor!).

- A *decrease* in your resting heart may indicate an improvement in your heart's health. Your heart has become more efficient at pumping blood. Congratulations!

Caution if it Hurts (You Can't Undo Years in Days)

"Don't Care How, I want it Now!"

~ Veruca Salt, Willy Wonka and the Chocolate Factory

You cannot undo years of accumulation in days. Have patience. If your knees, or any other part of you, are in pain during or after exercise, you may be going at it a little too hard or your body may be in the wrong position for the movement. Pain is your body's caution light. Soreness, on the other hand, can be expected as you strengthen your knees and other parts of your body.

Everyone wants a magic pill to immediately take care of weight loss or body aches and pains, but it doesn't exist. Work into your new routine and habits slowly. Master one or two things before moving on. If you follow the Healthy Knees plan, you should see progress in just a few weeks and make significant changes within months.

Too Much: The Warning Signs

All of our Healthy Knees Cycling Coaches are trained to watch for warning signs when you cycle. However, we want you to be aware, as well.

If ever you feel dizzy or nauseous while exercising, back down on your intensity and/or stop your activity. You have pushed too hard. Again, as an athlete, you'll learn what is "normal" for you. If you ever feel you are outside of that zone, please seek medical assistance immediately.

Do not ignore:

1) Chest pain

2) Shortness of breath (a change in your normal pattern)

3) Nausea

4) Dizziness, fainting, loss of consciousness

5) Fatigue (a change from your normal pattern)

6) Heart palpitations – abnormally high or irregular heartbeats

Now you are ready to hop on your well-adjusted bike and use proper body position while putting energy into your pedals. It is a good idea to have a feeling of how-hard-is-hard for you. You can begin to push that a little and measure how quickly your heart rate recovers or going from feeling like you are working hard to feeling like it is easy. You don't need to go all out and suffer every time you exercise. Instead, I recommend pushing your levels of comfort a little bit more each time you cycle. Your knees and your heart get in better shape and thank you!

CHAPTER 8

6 HEALTHY KNEES STARTER CYCLING WORKOUTS

It is time to ride! In these starter workouts, you'll focus on practicing the fundamentals and building stamina and strength. If you haven't been cycling much before now, keep in mind your hiney will be a little sore. That is normal. It takes just a couple of weeks to get used to the saddle. Be sure you are in a neutral hip position and you feel the pressure at the back of the saddle, not the nose of the saddle. For the best results, ride two or three times per week.

The six workouts provided here give you a good foundation for building strength and "oiling" your creaky knee hinges. Full size 8.5" X 11" printouts are available on our website at **www.HealthyKneesBook.com/ resources** and are also available as a follow-along video series available at **www.HealthyKneesBook.com/Videos**

These six workouts were designed to be completed in order. It is best to do two or three workouts per week; once per week is not quite enough if you are serious about making progress. If you are just starting out, give yourself a day recovery in between the cycling workouts (this is a good day to do your strength and core training!)

- If any one of the workouts is too long for you: That's OK, we all need to start somewhere. Simply do as much as you can, then stop. Repeat the workout until you can complete it, then move on to the next.

- If the workout is not quite enough: If you can easily complete the workout and want more, simply repeat one or more of the interval sets to increase the time.

Healthy Knees Cycling: 6 Fundamental Workouts

#1   Form Foundations (30 min)

#2   Pedal Fundamentals (30 min)

#3   Hills, Valleys, and Surges (32 min)

#4   Strength and Endurance 101 (35 min)

#5   Power Builder 1:1 (37 min)

#6   Rolling Hills (36 min)

Healthy Knees Cycling #1: Form Foundations   Total Time: 30 minutes

Focus: Body Position, Pedal Speed, Pedal Tension
Purpose: To build understanding and body mechanics to support healthy knees.
Rate of Perceived Exertion (RPE) Zones: Z1 = Easy, Z2 = Moderate, Z3 = Hard,
Z4 = Very Hard, Z5= Max Effort

Interval Time (min)	Focus	Cue	RPM	RPE/HR Zone
4:00	Warm Up	Easy spin. Add enough tension so you feel you are pushing against something	75+	1
1:00	Body Check #1 Foot Position	Foot Position: No Tippy Toes! Foot should be parallel to the floor with up to 20 degree heel lift.	75+	2
1:00	Body Check #2 Knee Position	Knee Position: Optimally, knees are parallel to bike or tucked in. Not flared out.	75+	2
1:00	Body Check #3 Sit Bones	Sit Bones: Feel your weight at the back of the saddle on your sit bones.	75+	2
1:00	Body Check #4 Flat Back, Relaxed Shoulders	Flat Back: Not arched or scooped. Shoulders: Inhale and raise shoulder to your ears; exhale and release all the tension in shoulders.	75+	2
1:00	Body Check #5 Al Dente Elbows	Elbows: soft with a slight bend. Not stick straight like uncooked pasta or too bendy like overcooked pasta.	75+	2
1:00	Body Check #6 Rolled Wrists	Rolled Wrists: Create a long line from your forearm to the top of your hand. No "cocked" wrists.	75+	2
6:00	RPM Pyramid	0:30 at each RPM. Take off tension, if necessary, to pedal at the higher speeds. 65-70-75-80-85-90-85-80-75-70-65-60.	65-90-60	2 - 3
2:00	Recovery	Easy spin!	75+	1
2:00	Tension Drill #1 Hold RPM steady	0:30 Light Tension 0:30 Medium Tension (add a gear or two) 0:30 Heavy Tension (add a gear or two) 0:30 Easy Recovery (take off some tension)	70	2 3 4 1
2:00	Tension Drill #2	Repeat above at new RPM.	75	Repeat
2:00	Tension Drill #3	Repeat above at new RPM.	80	above
6:00	Cool Down	Easy spin, bring your heart rate down.	75-90	1

Healthy Knees Cycling #2: Pedal Fundamentals   Total Time: 30 minutes

Focus: Pedal Stroke, Pedal Speed, Pedal Tension

Purpose: To continue to build body awareness and develop body mechanics to support healthy knees.

Rate of Perceived Exertion (RPE) Zones: Z1 = Easy, Z2 = Moderate, Z3 = Hard, Z4 = Very Hard, Z5= Max Effort

Interval Time (min)	Focus	Cue	RPM	RPE/ HR Zone
5:00	Warm Up	Easy spin. Add enough tension so you feel you are pushing against something.	75+	1
5:00	Pedal Stroke	Practice each part of the Pedal Stroke: Downstroke, Bottomstroke, Upstroke, Topstroke 2:00: Alternate 0:30 each 2:00: Alternate 0:30 each 1:00: Alternate 0:15 each	75- 85	2
2:00	Recovery	Easy spin.	75+	1
2:30	Pedal Speed Interval	Increase RPM every 0:30. If you can, leave your tension as is. If necessary, release some tension so you can reach the RPM.	70-75-80-85-90	2-3
2:30	Pedal Speed Interval	Repeat above.	70-75-80-85-90	2-3
2:00	Recovery	Easy spin.	75+	1
2:00	Tension Drill #1	Hold RPM steady 0:30 Light Tension 0:30 Medium Tension (add a gear or two) 0:30 Heavy Tension (add a gear or two) 0:30 Easy Recovery (take off some tension)	70	2 3 4 1
2:00	Tension Drill #3	Repeat above at new RPM.	75	Repeat above
2:00	Tension Drill #2	Repeat above at new RPM.	80	
5:00	Cool Down	Easy spin, bring your heart rate down.	75-90	1

Healthy Knees Cycling #3: Hills, Valleys, and Sur

Total Time: 32 minutes

Focus: Refining Pedal Speed and Building Power

Purpose: To continue to develop muscular control and begin to build strength and power.

Rate of Perceived Exertion (RPE) Zones: Z1 = Easy, Z2 = Moderate, Z3 = Hard, Z4 = Very Hard, Z5= Max Effort

Interval Time (min)	Focus	Cue	RPM	RPE/ HR Zone
5:00	Warm Up	Easy spin. Add enough tension so you feel you are pushing against something.	75+	1
0:30	Power	Hold RPM, add tension so it is very hard.	80	4
1:00	Warm Up	Easy Spin.	75+	1
0:30	Pedal Speed	Add 10 RPM to wherever you are. Pedal Faster!	85+	3
1:00	Warm Up	Easy Spin.	75+	2
4:00	Pedal Stroke Try to pedal a bigger circle than your pedals allow.	Practice each part of the Pedal Stroke: Downstroke, Bottomstroke, Upstroke, Topstroke 2:00: Alternate 0:30 each 1:00: Alternate 0:15 each 1:00: Put it all together!	80-90	2
1:00	Recover	Easy Spin.	75+	1
2:00	Increase RPM	Every 0:30, add 5 RPM.	80, 85, 90, 95	3
1:30	Decrease RPM	Every 0:30, decrease 5 RPM.	90, 85, 80	3
2:00	Recover	Easy Spin!	75+	1
2:00	Decrease RPM	Every 0:30, decrease 5 RPM, add Tension to make it harder like the hill is getting steeper.	90, 80, 70, 65	3
1:30	Increase RPM	Every 0:30, increase 5 RPM, take off a little tension like the hill is getting more gradual.	70, 80, 90	3
2:00	Recover	Easy Spin!	75+	1
3:00	Surge Intervals	Repeat 1:00 Interval Set 3X 0:45 hold 70 RPM; 0:15 Pedal Faster to 90 RPM Do not change tension, work to pedal faster!	70/90	2/4
5:00	Cool Down	Easy spin, bring your heart rate down.	75-90	1

Healthy Knees Cycling #4: Cycle Strength and Endurance 101 Total Time: 35 minutes

Focus: Intervals that build strength

Purpose: Stronger muscles and more stamina! Using our good cycling technique to hold longer intervals to begin to build strength and endurance

Rate of Perceived Exertion (RPE) Zones: Z1 = Easy, Z2 = Moderate, Z3 = Hard, Z4 = Very Hard, Z5= Max Effort

Interval Time (min)	Focus	Cue	RPM	RPE/ HR Zone
5:00	Warm Up	Easy spin. Add enough tension so you feel you are pushing against something.	75+	1
0:30	Power	Hold RPM, add tension so it is very hard.	80	4
1:00	Warm Up	Easy Spin.	75+	1
0:30	Pedal Speed	Add 10 RPM to wherever you are. Pedal Faster!	85+	3
1:00	Warm Up	Easy Spin.	75+	2
2:00	½ Rotation Track Stand	With pedals stopped and feet parallel to ground, transition from seated to standing. Pedal 1/2 stroke to switch position of feet. Return to seated. Repeat, starting with other foot.	0	2
2:00	1 Rotation Track Stand	Same as above, but make full rotation of pedals. Start with opposite foot each time you stand.	0	2
2:00	Standing Drills	Alternate 0:15 seated/0:15 standing and pedaling. Weight should be in your feet, not your hands. If you feel you are not yet ready for this, continue with the track stand and rotation drills.	60-70	2
2:00	Recover	Easy Spin!	75+	1
5:00	Surge Intervals	Repeat Interval Set 5X 0:45 hold 70 RPM 0:15 Pedal Faster to 90 RPM Do not change tension, work to pedal faster!	70/90	2/4
2:00	Recover	Easy Spin!	75+	1
2:30	Seated Climb	Add Tension and slow by 5 RPM every 0:30.	90-85-80-75	4
2:00	Downhill	Easy Spin.	85+	1
2:30	Seated Climb	Add Tension and slow by 5 RPM every 0:30.	90-85-80-75	4
5:00	Cool Down	Easy spin, bring your heart rate down.	75-90	1

Healthy Knees Cycling #5: Power Builder 1:1

Total Time: 37 minutes

Focus: Intervals with ratio of 1 work to 1 rest

Purpose: Developing muscular strength, stamina, and power

Rate of Perceived Exertion (RPE) Zones: Z1 = Easy, Z2 = Moderate, Z3 = Hard, Z4 = Very Hard, Z5= Max Effort

Interval Time (min)	Focus	Cue	RPM	RPE/ HR Zone
5:00	Warm Up	Easy spin. Add enough tension you feel you are pushing against something.	75+	1
0:30	Power	Hold RPM, add tension so it is very hard.	80	4
1:00	Warm Up	Easy Spin.	75+	1
0:30	Pedal Speed	Add 10 RPM to wherever you are. Pedal Faster!	85+	3
1:00	Warm Up	Easy Spin.	75+	2
4:00	Pedal Stroke	Practice Downstroke, Bottomstroke, Upstroke, Topstroke 2:00 with 0:30 each pedal stroke 1:00 with 0:15 each pedal stroke 1:00 Put it all together! Pressure all the way around the pedal.	75-85	2-3
2:00	Recover	Easy Spin!	75+	1
2:00	1:1 Interval	1:00 Work Hard; 1:00 Recover.	85+	3/1
4:00	2:2 Interval	2:00 Work Hard; 2:00 Recover.	80	3/1
6:00	3:3 Interval	3:00 Work Hard; 3:00 Recover.	75	3/1
4:00	2:2 Interval	2:00 Work Hard; 2:00 Recover.	80	3/1
2:00	1:1 Interval	1:00 Work Hard; 1:00 Recover.	85+	3/1
5:00	Cool Down	Easy spin, bring your heart rate down.	75-90	1

Healthy Knees Cycling #6: Rollers   Total Time: 36 minutes

Focus: Drills for Hills

Purpose: Developing strength and force

Rate of Perceived Exertion (RPE) Zones: Z1 = Easy, Z2 = Moderate, Z3 = Hard, Z4 = Very Hard, Z5= Max Effort

Interval Time (min)	Focus	Cue	RPM	RPE/ HR Zone
5:00	Warm Up	Easy spin. Add enough tension so you feel you are pushing against something.	75+	1
0:30	Power	Hold RPM, add tension so it is very hard.	80	4
1:00	Warm Up	Easy Spin.	75+	1
0:30	Pedal Speed	Add 10 RPM to wherever you are. Pedal Faster!	85+	3
1:00	Warm Up	Easy Spin.	75+	2
2:00	½ Rotation Track Stand	With pedals stopped and feet parallel to ground, transition from seated to standing. Pedal 1/2 stroke to switch position of feet. Return to seated. Repeat, starting with other foot.	0	2
2:00	1 Rotation Track Stand	Same as above, but make full rotation of pedals. Start with opposite foot each time you stand.	0	2
2:00	Standing Drills	Alternate 0:15 seated/0:15 standing and pedaling. Weight should be in your feet, not your hands. If you feel you are not yet ready for this, continue with the track stand and rotation drills.	60-70	2
2:00	Recover	Easy Spin!	85+	1
5:00	Rolling Hill Interval	1:30 Flat Road. 2:30 Climb. 1:00 Descent.	85-90 75-80 90+	3 4 1
5:00	Rolling Hill Interval	1:30 Flat Road. 2:30 Climb. 1:00 Descent.	85-90 75-80 90+	3 4 1
5:00	Rolling Hill Interval	1:30 Flat Road. 2:30 Climb. 1:00 Descent.	85-90 75-80 90+	3 4 1
5:00	Cool Down	Easy spin, bring your heart rate down.	75-90	1

CHAPTER 9

BUT WAIT! THERE IS MORE… STRENGTH, CORE, STRETCHING

Reducing knee pain and strengthening your knees takes more than just cycling. Cycling is the lubricant for your knees and strengthens them in many ways. For the best chance at keeping your knees the strongest and healthiest they can be, add strength training, core exercises, and stretching. Why?

If you have a muscle weakness, your body is incredibly good at finding a way to compensate. Compensation, however, can lead to other problems by over-using the muscles that are taking on more work. Pretty soon you might have knots and pain in other places. Or find you are always favoring your calf or have a nagging hip injury. The way to keep your knees in tune is by strengthening all of the muscles that help your knees do their work.

The exercises I provide are, by no means, an exhaustive list. They are my bare bones "must haves" for taking care of your knees. They are just the very top crystal of ice in a very large iceberg. There are so many awesome exercises for leg strength, core strength, and stretching!

8 Essential Strength Moves to Support Healthy Knees

To keep your knees strong and stable, it is important to strengthen not only the muscles connecting to the knee, but also the muscles controlling leg movement.

There are many, many exercises to support healthy knees. These are my top recommendations (which can be performed starting with bodyweight, only) to help you both on and off the bike. Once you have mastered the movement with good form, go to the next advancement in the progression. If you are able to complete all of the progressions with good form, start adding challenges (such as adding resistance with bands, dumbbells, or a cable machine).

Work up to a set of 12-15 repetitions per movement. You should not feel any knee pain in the process.

The number one "DON'T" of exercises for healthy knees: in any of the moves, do not allow your knee to pass in front of the toes of your foot when doing a squat or lunge move. To avoid this, reposition your hips farther back like you are going to sit in a chair. It's ok, stick out your booty!

There is more help than I could fit in this book. Print out your own copy of these exercises with pictures **www.HealthyKneesBook.com/ Resources**. If you want more guidance on exactly how to do the moves, check out the video at **www.HealthyKneesBook/Bonus**.

HK Strength #1: Squat Progression (Front of thigh Quadriceps muscles, back of thigh Hamstrings muscles, hip extension Gluteus muscles)

Healthy Knees Tip: Make sure your knees do not pass in front of your toes. Stick out your booty! Be sure your feet are pointed straight ahead for good knee alignment.

Squat Start: Wall Sit

Squat Advance 1: Supported Squat: Ball on Wall

Squat Advance 2: Supported Squat: Suspension Training Squat

Squat Advance 3: Partial Squat: Squat to Chair, Arms Raised

Squat Advance 4: Body Weight Squat

More Squat Variations: Add weights or change your stance (narrow, wide, sumo, lift leg)

HK Strength #2: Step Ups (Front of thigh Quadriceps muscles and hip extension Gluteus muscles)

Healthy Knees Tip: Make sure your knee does not pass in front of your toes. Stick out your booty! Start with body weight only, advance your position, and then add weights.

Step Ups Start: Side Facing Step ups

Step Ups Advance 1: Side Facing Step ups with squat

Step Ups Advance 2: Add weights

HK Strength #3: Seated Leg Extension (primarily front of thigh Quadriceps muscles)

Healthy Knees Tip: While seated with the majority of your thigh supported by the chair, start this exercise with one foot off the ground and leg bent at 45 degrees. Straighten your leg to be parallel with the floor, and return to 45 degrees. Do not touch your foot to the ground until you have finished your repetitions. Only work from the 45-degree angle to full extension, then repeat. Add weights as you get stronger.

Seated Leg Extension Start: Body Weight only

Seated Leg Extension Advance: Add Weights (ankle weight)

HK Strength #4: Outer Thigh Side Leg Lift Progressions (Outer Thigh Abductor muscles)

Healthy Knees Tip: If you feel discomfort in your knee with a straight leg, try bending your knee just a bit and as you build strength and stability in your knee, you may eventually be able to do this series of exercises with a straight leg. Do *not* shift your hip as you lift your leg.

Only lift your leg as high as you can while keeping your hips stable and aligned. This exercise helps with strength and hip mobility.

Start Side Leg Lift: Standing (chair or wall support)

Advance 1: Standing with Band at Knees

Advance 2: Side Lying Leg Lift

Advance 3: Side Lying Partial Side Plank Leg Lift

Advance 4: Side Lying Full Plank Leg Lift

HK Strength #5: Inner Thigh Leg Lift Progressions (inner thigh - adductor muscles)

Healthy Knees Tip: If you feel discomfort in your knee with a straight leg, try bending your knee just a bit and as you build strength and stability in your knee, you may eventually be able to do this series of exercises with a straight leg. Be cautious in adding weight to this move; try a band above your knees. The additional lateral stress in your knee may cause discomfort. If it does, do not add weight.

Start Inner Thigh: Standing Adduction

Advance 1: Side Lying Adduction (bottom leg lift)

HK Strength #6 Calf Raises (Foot extension and flexion muscles in your calf and front of shin)

Healthy Knees Tip: You may find this exercise more challenging on your weaker leg. Balance may be difficult. Hold on to a chair or the wall; placing your hands on your hips may improve balance. When advancing, use control! Overstretching your Achilles tendon may lead to other issues.

Start Calf Raises: Both Feet on Floor

Advance 1: Both Feet on Step (dropping heel)

Advance 2: Single Leg on Floor

Advance 3: Single Leg (on step)

HK Strength #7: Donkey Kick (back of thigh knee flexion hamstring muscles and hip extension gluteus muscles)

Traditionally this move is done on the floor, but I know some may have problems with kneeling. For all options, do *not* engage (arch) your lower back when lifting your leg. Make the movement from your hip only.

Start Donkey Kick: Standing

Advance 1: Tabletop Bent Knee

Advance 2: Tabletop Leg extension

HK Strength #8: Good Mornings (Back of thigh Hamstring muscles for knee flexion and hip extensor Gluteus muscles)

From a standing position with feet about shoulder width apart and a flat back, hinge forward at your hips until you feel a stretch in your hamstring (but upper body no lower than parallel to the floor), pause, and return to standing.

Start Good Mornings: Both Feet on the floor with hands on hips.

Advances: Change your center of balance to make this move more challenging. 1) Move your hands to your chest, 2) Clasp your hands at the back of your head with elbows wide, 3) Add weight by holding a barbell resting on your shoulders behind your neck.

Alternative Move Balance Challenge: Single Leg (reach leg and opposite arm)

7 Essential Core Moves to Support Healthy Knees

Did you know your core strength is an important component to maintaining healthy knees? It all goes back to the kinetic chain with the parts of our body, not as independent, but linked together. When one part is weak or injured, it may invariably affect other connected bones and muscles.

A strong core helps support a healthy skeletal structure in your back and hips which affect your leg alignment. And vice versa: a weakness in your leg can affect your hips and back. A strong core helps prevent this.

Almost all of these exercises require you to get on the floor. If this is too difficult for you, try doing them on your bed. While the bed is not ideal because it is soft, you still gain benefit from the exercises.

Each exercise is listed with a "Start". Only advance once you have mastered this first step and can repeat it with good form for 12 repetitions. It does you no good to proceed if you cannot sustain good form for the duration of the move.

See all of the pictures with a printable version at
www.HealthyKneesBook.com/Resources.
See a video demonstrating the moves at

www.HealthyKneesBook.com/Bonus.

HK Core #1: Bird Dog Progressions

If the start position on hands and knees does not work for you, try doing this move standing. You'll still get some of the benefits! As you lift your leg behind you, engage your glute (butt) and only lift as high as you can without arching your back. If you don't feel like you are doing this right, try poking yourself in the butt of the lifting leg and making that muscle tense.

Start: In tabletop position (on hands and knees with a flat back) extend one arm without shifting your hips. Next, extend one leg without shifting your hips. When you can do this for both arms and both legs without shifting your hips, go to Advance 1. Note: You can do this exercise to some extent while standing.

Advance 1: Lift and extend (reach!) opposite arm and leg without shifting your hips. Hold, return to tabletop. Alternate with the other side. When you can do this for both combos of arm/leg, go to Advance 2.

Advance 2: Add in an elbow to knee crunch. After you extend and reach your arm and leg, bring your knee and elbow together under your belly for a crunch. Tighten your abdominal muscles as you do this: pull your belly in like you are zipping up a tight pair of pants.

HK Core #2: Back Extension Progressions

Start: Lying prone on your belly (face down), place your hands on the floor by your shoulders. Use your hands to support (not push) as you lift your shoulders and chest off the ground. Keep your head in a neutral position. Only rise about eight inches – try *not* to engage your glute muscles (your bottom).

Advance 1: Place your hands under your forehead and only use the muscles of your lower back to lift off the floor.

Advance 2: ½ Superman Extend your arms while facing down. Lift one arm and opposite leg about 8 inches off the floor. Hold for two counts. Switch arm and leg combo.

Advance 3: Superman! Extend both arms and legs and reach as you lift your shoulders and chest off the ground

Advance 4: Super Swimmer! While your arms and legs are extended and your shoulders and chest are lifted off the floor, flutter your arms and legs for about 10 seconds or more as you build strength.

HK Core #3: Sit-Up Progressions

Crunch Start: Lying supine on the floor (face up) with your knees bent and feet as close to your hiney as you can get them, put your hands on the floor by your hips and lift your shoulders and upper back off the floor as you slide your fingertips toward your hips. Engage your abdominals like you are pulling in your belly to zip up your pants and sliding your ribcage toward your hips.

Crunch Advance 1: Do the same movement, but place your hands on your chest.

Reverse Crunch: Start in the same position, with hands on the floor by your hips and knees bent. Without changing the bend in your knees, bring your knees toward your chest lifting your feet off the floor.

Double Crunch: With your hands behind your head for support (not to pull), do both the crunch and reverse crunch at the same time: bring your bent knees toward your chest as you crunch your chest toward your knees.

HK Core #4: Twist Progressions

Waiter's Tray Start: Standing with your elbows pinned to your sides, your forearms parallel to the floor, and palms facing in, keep your hips directed forward and twist at the waist (also rotating your shoulders) to the right and left.

Waiter's Tray Advance: Add a dumbbell or medicine ball held between your hands.

Bicycle Crunch

Lie flat on the floor with your lower back pressed and feeling like you are pulling your navel toward your spine. With your hands behind your head, lift a shoulder blade off the ground as you bring your elbow toward the opposite bent knee. Now, alternate! Think "bicycle" with your legs, rotating each opposite elbow toward your knee as it comes to your chest. Hover your extended leg over the floor but try not to touch the floor. No need to "sprint" with your legs. It is better to do this more slowly with intention. Be sure *not* to pull on your head or neck with the support of your hands. Vary going super slow and a moderate pace.

Bicycle Crunch Standing Option: If lying on the floor for this move is too much for you, try it standing up! Place your hands on your head with your elbows wide, lift opposite knee to elbow, alternate.

HK Core #5 Side Bend Progressions

Side Bend Start: Body Weight Only

Standing erect with your hands on the sides of your thighs, bend at the waist to the right, sliding your fingertips toward your knee. Keep your body in the same plane – as if you are in a toaster and would get burned if you tipped either way. Alternate side to side, with a pause at the top so momentum does not carry you from side to side.

Side Bend Advance 1: Same movement, but move your hands from your thighs to your head with your elbows high to the sides. Bring your elbow toward your hip and keep your body in the same plane.

Side Bend Advance 2: Add one dumbbell

Hold one dumbbell at your thigh and your free hand rests on the outside of your other thigh. Using your oblique (side) muscles, bend toward the free hand, sliding your free hand down your thigh. Use control in both directions! Complete your set on one side. Switch your dumbbell to the other hand and do your second set.

HK Core #6: Leg Lift Progressions

Start Scissor Kick: Lying on the ground supine (face up), place your hands just underneath your hips. Raise both legs straight so your heels are pointing to the ceiling. Keep one leg still and lower the other to just above the floor. Hold for a beat, and then switch legs.

If you cannot lie on the floor or your bed for this move, try it while standing. Keep your body erect (no leaning forward or backward) and keep your leg as straight as possible. Lift your leg as high in front of you as you can without shifting your upper body. Complete one set on one leg, then switch to the other.

Advance 1 Double Leg Lift: Start in the same position. Lower both legs to the floor at the same time, hover above the floor, and rise back up toward the ceiling.

Advance 2 Flutter Kick: Start in the same position, lower both feet to about 12 inches off the ground and flutter kick for 10 seconds or more.

Advance 3 Heel Drive: Start in the same position, now lift your hips off the ground as you drive your heels toward the ceiling. Do this motion with as much lift and control as you can. Try not to swing your legs as you lift toward the ceiling.

HK Core #7: Hip Bridge Progressions

Start Hip Bridge: Lying supine (face up) with your feet as close to your bottom as you can and your hands palms down on the floor by your hips,

1) Engage your core (tighten your belly)

2) Squeeze your glutes (clench your butt)

3) Lift your hips up to form a straight bridge from your shoulders to your knees. Hold for a count or two, tap your bottom down, and repeat.

Advance 1 Marching Hip Bridge: Start in the hip lifted position, "march" your feet. Lift one leg off the floor with the knee in the same position (do not bend more or less) and alternate marching. Keep your hips stable! Clench your glutes! Do not let one side of your hips lift or drop.

Advance 2 Single Leg Hip Bridge: In the supine start position, straighten one leg so your thighs are parallel and one foot is off the floor. Hold your leg extended, clench the glute of the leg with your foot on the ground and press up into the bridge position. Be aware of your hips! Do not let one side lift or drop as you press into the bridge. Tap down and repeat same side.

5 Essential Stretches to Support Healthy Knees

These five essential stretches for cyclists help your knees (and body) stay limber. If you have a balance issue, please hold on to something! Sometimes simply touching your hands on your own body or pressing your hands together help you balance better.

To see pictures of all the core moves with a printable version, go to
www.HealthyKneesBook.com/Resources.
If you would like to see the moves demonstrated,
check out the video at **www.HealthyKneesBook.com/Bonus**

HK Stretch #1: Calf

While standing, take a large step backward with one foot. With both feet pointing forward, keep your weight on your bent front leg. Bring the heel of your back leg toward the floor for a calf stretch with a straight leg. Take in a deep breath, raise your arms and eyes to the ceiling, exhale and bring your arms back to your sides. Bring your feet together and repeat on the other side.

HK Stretch #2: Hamstring

While standing, step one foot forward and with your forward foot, leave your heel on the ground, straighten your leg, and raise your toes. Transfer your weight to your back leg with knee slightly bent and a flat back, hinge forward at your hips (keep your hands on your hips or, if you need help with balance hold onto your bike or a wall or rest your hands on your legs). Take in a deep breath and as you exhale, stretch a little more and lift your toe even higher. Step back to standing and repeat on the other side.

HK Stretch #3: Glutes

While standing, bring one knee to your chest and give it a hug. Cross your knee over your belly and feel the stretch in your glutes. Return to center, lower your leg and repeat on the other side.

HK Stretch #4: Quads

Depending on your knee range of motion, you may need help with this one.

No Assist Quad Stretch: *This is only for you if you have the ability to fully flex your knee. If you have limited range of motion, use one of the assists.*

While standing, bring your heel toward your bottom and grab onto your ankle. Your knees should be side by side and body erect. If you go through any gymnastics to do this or your knee is sticking out to the side, or if you are bending one way or the other, *don't!* Use one of the assists, below.

Quad Stretch Assist with a Towel: Instead of grabbing your ankle as in the stretch above, hold onto a small towel wrapped around your ankle. Use proper alignment with knees side by side, hips pressed forward, standing tall.

Quad Stretch Assist with a Chair: Standing in front of a chair like you are going to sit down, raise one leg up behind you, and rest your foot on the chair. You may need to bend the leg you are standing on to deepen the stretch.

HK Stretch #5: Hip Flexors

Hip flexors are the muscles responsible for lifting your thigh, and get tight with cyclists and anyone who sits for long periods of time.

Hip Flexor Assist with a Chair: Before you do this, make sure your chair is not going to slide! Face your chair, feet about 3 feet away from it. Place one foot on the chair and sink down into the groin stretch. You may need to move your foot on the floor a little farther back to feel it. Inhale and as you exhale, relax, and stretch a little deeper.

Hip Flexor on the floor:

Get into a plank position and step one foot to the outside of one of your hands. Let your hips sink down into the stretch, feeling your hips open up. Deepen this stretch by lifting the hand (by your foot) toward the ceiling while rotating your upper body to a side facing position. Look up at your hand. Return your hand to the inside of your foot, step your foot back to plank and repeat on the other side.

CHAPTER 10

OTHER KINDS OF PAIN RELIEF: BRACES, INJECTIONS, TAPING, ROLLING, and DRUGS

Your path to healthier knees has some ups and downs. As you stress your knees with more movement, they may get a little achy while they become stronger. This should be short in duration. There is a difference between soreness and pain: soreness goes away in a day or two, but pain persists. At some point you may cry "Uncle" and want some help with managing your pain. I understand. I've been there too. In fact, I've tried some form of all of the methods below (except stem cell injections only because I haven't felt I've needed to try it yet and they are quite pricey.) I massage my scars daily, regularly use the kinesiology tape when I am active, and I foam roll my legs two or three times per week. This list of common pain relief methods for knees is arranged in order of simple solutions to more complex.

I view surgery as the last resort. All efforts should first be made to strengthen your supporting muscles and joint before heading to the knife. However, there may be a time where you, too, consider surgery when weighing your quality of life versus your pain.

When your pain begins to reduce your activity, you can end up in a bad spiral: reduced activity results in muscle loss, muscle loss adds to weakness, weakness adds to pain, and round and down you go.

It is time to stop this crazy cycle! Here are a few options for external sources of pain reduction (in addition to cycling, strength training, and stretching). The emphasis should be on you getting as strong as you can so you can live life to the fullest!

Give your Scars Some Love

A scar should not limit your joint mobility. Scars are formed when your skin tissue is knitting itself back together. Your body is very smart because it wants to prevent trauma to the area again so scars want to be very stable. To do this, the scar tissue sends 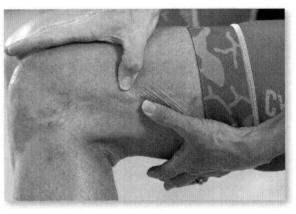 out fibers (like roots) to stabilize the whole area. The scar fibers may reach into the underlying tissues and cause adhesions or little sticking points, and this can be painful. Scars can get lumpy because of the buildup of the scar tissue underneath.

To prevent this and keep your skin mobile around your scar, manipulate the scar area. As soon as the scar has primarily healed (no more scabs), begin to very gently massage it. The pressure of your finger on your scar should be the equivalent of holding a quarter on your finger. Very light pressure!

- With one finger, massage back and forth across the scar.
- With two fingers on either side of the scar move up and down and in opposite directions.
- With one finger, massage in circles over the scar
- Eventually, you can "pick-up" the scar and roll along its length.

The tissue around the massage area may feel pinch-y or tingly. That is OK and shows scar tissue "roots" are breaking up.

See the demonstration of scar manipulation with the video at **www.HealthyKneesBook.com/Resources**.

What about vitamin E? There is a popular belief vitamin E oil rubbed into your skin may help scar tissue heal. However, a (1999)[15] study showed topically applied Vitamin E does not help improve the appearance of surgical scars, may actually be detrimental to appearance, and may lead to an incidence of contact dermatitis.

How I feel about scars...I have some very large scars on one of my legs and smaller ones on my other. I was out to lunch one day with a new acquaintance and I happened to be wearing a skirt. She saw the scars on my leg and said "You are so brave to wear a skirt." I was a little taken back by this comment because my scars are a part of who I am. I am not ashamed of them at all. My scars simply tell my story of the life I have lived. I hope you, too, can find peace with your scars.

Foam Rolling for Myofascial Release

Myofascial release (or foam rolling/trigger point release) was once only used by professional coaches and therapists for their athletes. However, this technique is available to all and I highly recommend you perform it on yourself regularly (several times per week).

Foam rolling is possibly the best restorative technique I have ever used. At first, it can be painfully uncomfortable. As you consistently use a roller, you should find relief. Your muscles feel renewed after

---

[15] Baumann MD, L. and Spencer MD MS, J. (1999) *The Effects of Topical Vitamin E on the Cosmetic Appearance of Scars*. 1999 American Society of Dermatologic Surgery. Retrieved 8/24/15 from **http://onlinelibrary.wiley.com/doi/10.1046/j.1524-4725.1999.08223.x/abstract?deniedAccessCusto misedMessage=&userIsAuthenticated=false**

you roll! Plus you'll reduce achy pain and knots. Foam rolling can help with muscle tension relief, increasing range of motion, preventing injury, and reducing or eliminating sticking points contributing to muscle imbalances.

Here is how it works: Fascia is a thin, elastic soft connective tissue that is intimately attached to your muscles. It is kind of like a tough silky casing around your muscles. It provides support and protection and helps your muscles glide against your skin. Your fascia can become "restricted," "impinged," or "adhered," creating taut bands of scar between skin and fascia. Inflammation can occur and the connective tissue can thicken, creating sore spots or knots.

Rolling helps to break up these sticking points to allow your underlying muscles and fascia to do their job and glide easier. Pay special attention to your quadriceps, Iliotibial band (IT band, the side of your leg), hamstring, and calf. There are many techniques to rolling, but the one I find most beneficial is to lie on the roller and start at the distal end of the muscle group (the point farther away from your core). Roll up about 4 inches, back 2 inches, up 4 inches, and back 2 inches, slowly creeping up your leg; reverse direction and roll, using the same method back to your starting point.

Kinesiology Taping

You've probably seen professional athletes sporting brightly colored tape on their arms, shoulders, or legs. This is not just for show, but is designed to alleviate pain or stress in a particular area. The tape is a self-adhesive, thin stretchy strip of woven cotton or synthetic fabric constructed to have the same elasticity as skin. The strip of tape bends and moves with skin without binding, constricting, or restricting movement.

Hypothetically, when applied to skin along muscles, ligaments, or tendons, the tape may give external support and allow for lymphatic drainage by microscopically lifting the skin away from the affected area. The theory is increased stability and lymphatic drainage may result in reduced inflammation.

Fad or Real? Does kinesio taping help with your knee pain? At about $20 per roll it is worth a try. I have found significant pain relief and support from taping. There is a growing body of evidence showing the benefits of pain relief and resulting increase in muscle power output. A study by Anandkumar et al. (2014)[16] used a double blind group of 40 people with knee arthritis between the ages of 45 and 60. The group was randomly allocated into either the experimental group (using KT tape with tension) or the control group (using KT tape without tension). The two groups were tested for isokinetic quadriceps torque and pain during movement. The results of their study group showed kinesiology tape is effective in improving muscle power and reducing pain in knee osteoarthritis.

If you are interested in using kinesiology tape, proper application is the key. Check with your doctor, physical therapist, or check with your gym for a trained taper. There are many tutorials available online as well.

Off-Loader Brace

An off-loader knee brace gently changes the alignment of your leg, redirecting your line of body weight to the healthiest side of the knee. A review of studies (2012)[17] showed an off-loading brace may be an effective way to reduce pain in an osteoarthritic knee. With reduced pain comes increased function and improved quality of life. The brace

---

[16] Anandkumar, S., Sudarshan, S., & Nagpal, P., (2014). **Efficacy of kinesio taping on isokinetic quadriceps torque in knee osteoarthritis: a double blinded randomised controlled study.** *Physiotherapy Theory and Practice: 10.3109/09593985.2014.896963*

[17] Feehan BS, N., Trexler CO, G., Barringer MS., W (2012) *The Effectiveness of Off-Loading Knee Orthoses in the Reduction of Pain in Medial Compartment Knee Osteoarthritis: A Systematic Review. American Academy of Orthotists & Prosthetists.* Retrieved on 8/24/15 from **http://www.oandp.org/jpo/library/2012_01_039.asp.**

might feel a bit bulky to wear but can be very effective in relieving pain especially during weight bearing activity.

Injections

Injections to relieve pain are given between the bones of the knee in the joint cavity (2014)[18]. This kind of injection is called intraarticular (IA). The most common injections are listed here in order of most common/effective to trial technologies. Recommendations for which type of injection (if any) may be best for you depend upon your joint condition, age, and weight.

Do they work? The only proven technology is corticosteroids. Others are still awaiting scientific proof of efficacy or, as in Hyaluronic Acid, have been proven ineffective. They've all had a variety of studies about effectiveness and the results range from placebo to very affective. My take is: it depends on the individual. While you may not respond to one type of treatment, another may work well. I figure if it gives you pain relief, it is better than the risks of an invasive procedure for a surgery.

Corticosterioids (e.g. Cortisone)

Corticosteroids help reduce inflammation through a complex action. They interrupt the inflammatory response at several levels which help reduce pain and may increase joint mobility. A cortisone shot usually includes corticosteroid medication and local anesthetic (2013)[19].

18 Ayhan, E, Kesmezacar, H., Akgun, I. (2014) *Intraarticular injections (corticosteroid, hyaluronic acid, platelet rich plasma) for the knee osteoarthritis.* World Journal of Orthopedics. Retrieved 8/24/15 from **http://www.ncbi.nlm.nih.gov/pmc/articles/PMC4095029/**.

19 Mayo Clinic (2013) *Cortisone Shots.* Retrieved 9/8/15 from **http://www.mayoclinic.org/tests-procedures/cortisone-shots/basics/definition/prc-20014455**.

Hyaluronic Acid or Viscosupplementation

It is called Viscosupplementation because the injection is proposed to enhance the viscosity of your synovial fluid. Hyaluronic Acid (HA) is a naturally-occurring component of synovial fluid (remember synovial fluid is like your joint oil). Viscosupplementation's role in synovial fluid is to enhance viscosity to act as a lubricant during slow joint movements and as an elastic shock absorber during rapid joint movement. It also helps reduce stress and friction on cartilage. Recent studies, however, are showing the HA injections do not add a lasting viscosity, are gone in a few days, and are now considered a placebo[20].

Platelet Rich Plasma (PRP)

Platelet Rich Plasma is prepared from the patient's own blood which is spun in a centrifuge to obtain a highly concentrated sample of platelets. The platelet solution is used to create a platelet gel rich in growth factors and bioactive molecules. These molecules are thought to act to reduce pain, inflammation, and improve function. PRP is a relatively new generation of bioactive treatments and is not yet widely used (and not yet proven).

Stem Cell

Stem cell injections are a promising bioactive technology and least widely used of the injections listed here. Mesenchymal stem cells, obtained from the patient's bone marrow or fat cells, have the potential to differentiate into any kind of cell, including cartilage and bone tissues. The premise is: stem cell application, both through IA injection or surgical implantation, may offer possible regenerative mechanisms to repair or possibly regenerate cartilage (2014)[21] and relieve pain.

---

[20]   Dr. Michael Thorpe, personal conversation, 11/25/15.

[21]   Pak, J., Lee, JH., Lee SH. (2014) *Regenerative Repair of Damaged Meniscus with Autologous Adipose Tissue-Derived Stem Cells.* US National Library of Medicine, National Institutes of Health. Retrieved on 9/8/15 from **http://www.ncbi.nlm.nih.gov/pmc/articles/PMC3925627/**

Drugs

Over the counter pain relieving drugs generally come in two forms: Non-Steroidal Anti-Inflammatory drugs ("NSAIDs") (such as ibuprofen, aspirin, naproxen sodium) and analgesics including acetaminophen known as Tylenol and Paracetamol among other brand names. These pain relievers come in many forms including coated and uncoated tablets, gel caps, caplets, and liquids.

Acetaminophen is primarily used to reduce headache pain and fever and is processed through the liver. NSAIDs, in addition to pain relief and fever reduction, also fight inflammation. NSAIDs are primarily processed through your kidneys and liver and may affect your gastrointestinal system. NSAIDs work by blocking an enzyme (cyclooxygenase or COX) that promotes inflammation, pain, and fever. However, COX-1 enzymes also protect the stomach and regulate blood clotting. When COX-1 is reduced by NSAIDs for an extended period, this may promote stomach ulcers and bleeding (2015)[22].

Should you take it? For Acetaminophen, NSAIDs, or other drugs, discuss with your doctor the pros and cons, risks, toxicity, and side effects.

---

[22] **MedicineNet.com** (Medically reviewed 1/30/15), retrieved on 10/25/15 from **www.medicinenet.com/ nonsteroidal_antiinlammatory_drugs/article.htm**

CHAPTER 11

POST-RIDE STORIES: THE LONG VIEW OF SUCCESS (CYCLING STORIES)

I wish you the very best in your knee health. I hope you use the information I've shared about cycling – the secrets in this book are only as good as the action you take. And remember, to see long lasting results, your effort needs to be ongoing. All the tips and secrets I've shared mean nothing if you try it a few times then stop. If you want meaningful changes, taking care of your knees (and body) need consistent, quality attention. I'd love to hear your stories of success and how you've been able to use cycling to feel better. Please send me an email with your story (and a picture!) to **Robin@HealthyKneesCycling.com**.

Please read on to enjoy a few stories of others.

Doug and Robin: "Bad Knees and a 10 Month Bicycle Journey Around the World"

(our story, as told by me!)

Traveling by bicycle is one of our favorite things to do as a couple. In 1990, even though walking (or especially going down stairs) did not feel very good, I could still cycle strongly. My husband and I wanted to have a grand adventure before we started a family of our own, so we quit our jobs and traveled around the world on our bicycles.

We had a very loose plan for this crazy adventure, but Doug wanted to start in New Zealand and I wanted to see Thailand. To save money, we planned on camping and cooking our own food. With guidebooks stowed and bicycle panniers fully packed we arrived fresh and ready to ride in Auckland, New Zealand.

Throughout our trip, we were having so much fun, our health was good, and our money held out so our three month adventure expanded to 10 months around the world. Here is a quick summary of our adventures:

- New Zealand (2 months): the roads were smooth and wide with nice shoulders, super friendly and welcoming people, beautiful countryside, hidden waterfalls, and plenty of sheep. Kiwi the fruit and Kiwi the bird (who loved to eat leather shoes tied to panniers, just saying.) Best campgrounds in the world.

  My left knee was already severely arthritic at this time. Riding my bike was great, but hiking, especially going downhill or big steps, was a painful challenge. Doug invented "elevator arm" to help me along, he always offered his shoulder or arm as an assist down the hills or steep steps (and still offers it to this day).

- Australia (1 month): we rode from Sydney to Brisbane but shipped our bikes from there to Darwin because the one main highway was not safe for us...I ended up blown off the road by the 4 trailer-long semi-trucks three times, crying we were going to get killed out there! Instead, we bought a bus pass and took a scuba diving certification course in the Great Barrier Reef. A good tradeoff, I think. Once we left Australia, we shipped our sleeping bags and bulky sweaters home since we would not be camping again (but we kept our tent and cookware just in case).

- Bali (1 week): narrow roads, with curious welcoming people. Monkeys and strange birds calling in the jungle. Tropical smells, banana pancakes, and tea in the mornings, simple living. I loved Bali.

Small world moment...we were walking along the unpopulated Penelokan rim road above the Batur caldera and a jeep pulled over. We thought, that's it, we are going to get mugged. Instead, out hopped Doug's roommate Stuart, from college and his brother John. What a welcome surprise!

- Singapore and Malaysia (3 weeks): Singapore was refreshing for its sense of order. We rode up the east coast of Malaysia and it was so hot we'd start at sun up and quit at about noon. It was hard to find enough water. We rode on the best roads in the world with their smoothness created from domestic rubber trees. People thought we were nuts for riding our bikes when the bus was so cheap.

- Thailand (3 weeks): no riding here. At that time, there was added risk in the southern part of the country. We took a train to Bangkok, stored the bikes at a hotel, and went north via train to trek in Chiang Mai.

  ~Originally we thought we might be flying home from here. But we were having so much fun (and our money was holding out!), we took our friend John's invitation to Hong Kong ~

- Hong Kong and a bit of China (2 weeks):

  We took the offer to visit John (from Bali) and indulged in a much-needed rest at his condominium in Hong Kong. We investigated the possibility of flying to Beijing to take the Trans-Mongolian train into Russia. Alas, we could not be guaranteed our bikes would travel on the same train as us. We scrapped that idea and simply flew into China to visit the beautiful Li River Valley out of Yangshuo where we rented the one-size, one-speed bikes of the people. Doug's knees were at his chin!

We revised our travel plans and invited our mothers to meet us in Europe. Since we were returning to cooler weather, we bought sweaters and sleeping bags in anticipation of camping again.

- England and Scotland (1 month): it rained or was windy or was both for everyday but three of the 30 days we were riding. We have (now) hilarious memories of nearly getting washed off a ferry exit ramp as waves crashed over the top; shrinking Doug's soaking wet poly-pro shirt in the dryer to doll size; and being generally wet and cold during the month of June. Thank goodness for warm pubs and good beer.
- Germany, Austria, and Switzerland with our mothers and my aunt (3 weeks):

  We met our mothers and my Auntie Tillie and stored our bikes while we travelled by car. It was a wonderful experience sharing this time together, but we were SO ready to leave the confinement of a car and get to back to the freedom of our two wheels.

- Germany, Austria, Over the Alps and into Yugoslavia (2 weeks):

  I thought I'd be ready for the three days of climbing through the Alps...but one day we had a 5K climb that was STEEP "obertauern" (meaning "over the top"). 5K? Sure, we can do anything for 5K!

  This was a definition of steep I had never known. It was so steep that I'd stop and let my burning quads have a break every ½ mile or so. When I started again, I had to zig zag across the highway while I worked to flip my pedal and slip my foot into the toe cage before I could head up the mountain (this was way before clipless pedals were common).

  It was an interesting time to travel in Yugoslavia. It was just months before the Yugoslav wars began (1991). We could feel the people's unrest and it was difficult to buy enough food at grocery stores to give us quality fuel. One big benefit of riding your bike all day is you get to/need to eat a lot. This is only a problem when you can't get food! We met some very interesting people and rode south through the hot, dry islands with steep rolling terrain and enticing swimming coves and campgrounds.

- Greece (3 weeks): Ah, lovely, hot Greece. My favorite memories are of campgrounds in olive groves, "undiscovered" beaches with crystal clear blue water and tropical fish, the warm generosity of the locals, and delicious food.

We logged over 5,000 miles in about 10 months. Given the chance, we'd do it all again.

Walt and Marilyn: "Family Bike Trip for ages 12 – 81"

What can a family that ranges from 12 years to 81 years of age do together. A bicycle trip, of course!

Walt and Marilyn Lonner are an adventurous couple who had an idea about an active family trip. Soon after Marilyn mentioned the idea to their son and daughter-in-law, the bicycle trip was booked from Passau, Germany to Vienna, Austria, following the famous bicycle path along the Danube. They worked with an Austrian company that helped them map their ride. Every day their gear would precede them from hotel

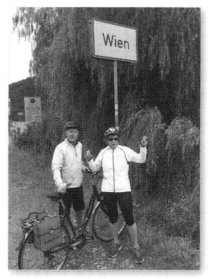

Walt and Marilyn reach Vienna!

to hotel. This gave Walt (81), Marilyn (78), their son and daughter-in-law plus two of their six granddaughters (ages 12 and 15) the chance to do something active together, make achievements every day, and experience travel in a whole new way.

The entourage rode an average of 30 to 35 miles per day, which they said was just right because it allowed time to take in the sights along the way and have lunch in picturesque villages. "I've been to Germany many times", said Marilyn, "and this was the first time in my life that I ever heard a real 'cuckoo'. The bird was right there in the tree as we pedaled by. It's what you can see and hear while you are riding a bike that is so wonderful."

Walt, a retired WWU professor, echoed similar sentiments "Every cyclist likes the freedom of movement, the ability to look around and hear and see things you'd never see from a car or even from one of those ubiquitous cruise ships seen up and down the Danube. Cruise ships provide plenty of food for the belly, but bicycling provides vitamins for the soul."

How did Walt and Marilyn prepare for this adventure? They both participated in Cycle Moles indoor cycling classes and rode their bikes outdoors, as they often do anyway, for 20 – 25 mile rides. Marilyn said that the techniques she learned in the cycling classes came in handy: "I could hear Robin's voice with reminders as I pedaled along the Danube 'push your sit bones to the back of the seat, roll your wrists, relax your shoulders'. I was not aware of biking techniques at all until I came to the Cycle Moles classes. I even shared these tips with my granddaughters to help them on their bikes."

Bob H.: "Taking on New Challenges at age 65"

Bob, now a retired ear, nose, throat physician, started running in the 1970s. He set big goals for himself, which he achieved: a sub 3-hour marathon (he ran 2:48), 10 miles in under 60 minutes, and a sub

5-minute mile (4:46 was his best). This all came to a halt at age 63 because of knee pain.

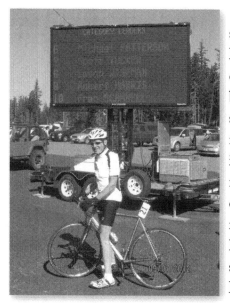
Bob's 9th place finish at Nationals 2012

About two years later, Bob started cycling at one of the Cycle Moles indoor classes. "Running caused swelling and kept me from basic movements like being able to squat. The more I cycled, the better my knees felt. After a couple of years into biking, it was no problem for my knees." Bob enjoyed the indoor cycling so much he expanded to ride outside. It wasn't long before he was entering events and gaining success. The first year he rode the Mt. Baker Hillclimb (24.5 miles uphill with 4,300+ foot gain), he smashed the record for 70 year olds of 3:05 by more than 40 minutes with a time of 2:14.

Cycling friends encouraged him to compete at the Nationals Masters Championship road race and in 2012, Bob placed 9th followed by an 8th place finish in 2015. "Cycling has been a wonderful thing for me. Not just for my knees, but for my retirement. I went from working full time in a successful career. The successes I've gained from biking fills the void of recognition I am missing from my work. I lost my wife last year and cycling helps to fill my time and gives me something to look forward to. I miss the people I used to work with and through cycling I've met new friends and have a new peer group. This is a very satisfying way to move into retirement."

Pat S. "Pain-Free Knees with Cycling!"

Letter from Pat in our Healthy Knees Cycle Camp

I think the healthy knees cycling camp is helping my knees and boosting my energy. Being part of a group makes the exercising more fun. Knowing that you, the leader (Robin), understand both human physiology and the physics of the bicycle makes me feel secure the settings are correct and the level of exertion is calculated to build strength and endurance without taxing the participant beyond safe limits.

I also love the music. It is sometimes very hard not to be singing along with every song. And the music most definitely acts to minimize my thoughts about discomfort (sort of like music in a dental office!).

Cannot think of anything I dislike. The first day, the seat was uncomfortable, but as the time has passed, the seat has become much more tolerable, even as we go for slightly longer periods of pedaling.

It has surprised and pleased me to discover I really like and enjoy the spinning bikes.... and I would definitely be interested in pursuing further healthy knees camps. Since we started this one, I have enjoyed completely knee-pain-free living --- and it seems only reasonable to me that if I continue to participate in similar camps, my knees and general health/energy can only benefit! Thank you very much for sharing your passion for cycling and your knowledge about healthy knees with all of us.

Nancy H.: "Ups and Downs with Steady Improvement"

I have experienced painful swelling in my right knee with a Baker's cyst that repeatedly leaked for several months. A cortisone injection brought relief, but only for about six weeks. Since beginning the cycling class I have had ups and downs - times my knee felt quite good and times when it really hurt. Inflammation and swelling have gone down for the most part. Pain and discomfort have been late in the day and during the night. My general health has been about the same. I have been doing cardio and strength training for 8-9 years. I am substituting cycling for an elliptical machine for cardio work two days each week. I am feeling very good about the stretching at the end of each class.

I like that I am using cycling as a long-term exercise plan to help deal with arthritic pain. I feel you both encourage and challenge all of us to keep improving. Your attention to cycle adjustments gives me the confidence I can proceed injury- free. Thank you for making this a growing, challenging and fun experience.

Thanks Robin for the steps you have taken to try to improve the quality of life for those suffering with painful knees!

Nancy W.: "Recovery from a Torn MCL"

Nancy tore her left MCL (medial collateral ligament) in November 2014. It was not diagnosed until late January so the healing process seemed slow. She was not in constant pain with her knee but "The times it hurts seems to be less often since I started the Healthy Knees class. My other main goal for the class was to increase my aerobic ability and I feel that has improved" says Nancy. "I finally figured out I needed an organized activity to get me started on my path to better health. This class was just what I needed; a way to get started back to being physically active."

Andy D. and Connie C.: "Touring on a Tandem"

Andy always liked bicycling and, even as a teen, rode bicycle tours and later a multi-state cross-country bicycle trip. For Connie, cycling was simply not a part of her life. Andy and Connie met on a cross-country ski trip some thirty years ago and have been married for twenty-eight years.

Their active lifestyle continued in a variety of ways with hiking, skiing, and bicycling. Their bicycle adventures started out on separate bikes with Andy (the stronger of the two) towing their two children in a bike trailer. Eventually, they tried a tandem bike and found it was a much better way for the two 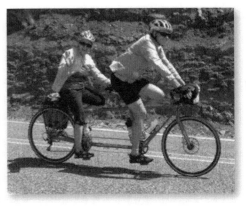 of them to ride together since they had a big disparity in their riding abilities. On a tandem, Connie felt good because she knew Andy wasn't waiting for her and since he has so much more cycling experience, it makes her feel safer. Andy loved it because they were able to stay together on their adventures and enjoy the time together even more.

Taking tandem trips with other couples was a joy. For their 25th anniversary they took a 12 day cycling trip to Languedoc, France with their tandem and a trailer, pulling their own luggage. What do they like most about cycling?

Connie says "I like the intimacy of a bike. It is slower, you take the backroads, and you are burning calories when you ride so you can fully enjoy the local cuisine. My husband and I both like to be active and doing it together on a tandem bike is fun...even when it rains! That always means a stop at a café for a nice hot cup of coffee."

Andy agrees and suggests if you cyclo-tour to carefully choose the region. "Be sure you know what you are getting into, whether it is flat and rolling terrain or steep hills. Our tandem trip to Turkey surprised us with painfully steep hills, but we made it. Train before you go and have the right gears on your bike for the terrain. Low gears save your knees."

Connie quit playing soccer a few years ago because of knee pain. She feels like she is healthier since starting cycling and enjoys the indoor training to get her ready for the outdoor experiences. Andy is shying away from running, but still enjoys hiking, playing tennis, and cycling. He attributes the hiking and cycling to making his knees strong.

George S.: "Knee Replacement and the Benefits of Cycling"

Letter from George:

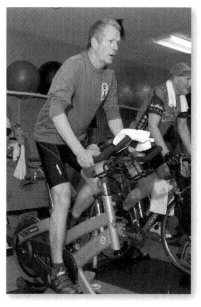

I totally agree with you cycling is great knee therapy.

After a lifetime of long distance running and so many injuries, the meniscus in my left knee was totally gone. Toward the end I tried to just run and later run-walk, but there was pain. Perhaps if I had switched earlier to nonimpact activities I could have prolonged use of my natural knee. At any rate, six years ago the pain was just too much. I couldn't walk any distance at all. I was in the first Cycle Moles class at the time and even that was too much. I had to stop. I had my knee replaced in March.

The first few weeks of rehabilitation were pretty rough. After eight weeks I was back to a normal riding routine. Four months after my knee replacement, I was able to ride the STP (200+ mile Seattle to Portland bicycle ride) with all of my family. After six years, I haven't had any problems with the replacement knee. I swim with the masters group three or four times a week and ride 2,500 to 3,000 miles a year. I had worried I might be wearing out the replacement knee, but a recent x-ray showed no visible signs of wear, and the surgeon thought it would likely last the rest of my life. What a relief.

Knee replacement is no fun, but in my case at least, it has allowed me to be just as active as when I had a healthy natural knee. I should also mention my right knee was down to about 50% of meniscus thickness when I had surgery. After six years of swimming and cycling it is still at 50% and hasn't given me any problems.

Larry G.: "Frayed Cartilage and No Pain on a Bike"
Larry's letter

While I'm thankful I've been active in sports and physical activity for most of my life, cycling has allowed me to stay fit and keep moving when my body isn't operating at top level.

At the Fresno City Tennis Championships in September of 2013, I lost the first round against a former tennis student. I then won two matches to reach the finals of the consolation bracket, my fourth match in two days. At the time I was 58, and not accustomed to playing more than one tournament match a day. I may have been the oldest player in the 4.5 division and the weather was hot, around 100 degrees, and even the morning temperatures were warm.

In the consolation final, my opponent played an aggressive game and made too many errors. My game was based on consistency and accuracy since I no longer have an edge in quickness or endurance. I played well, but I had to move quickly throughout the match and in the second set, I felt a distinct twinge in my left knee. I was worried the knee pain would get worse, but I was able to win 6-2, 6-3 in a match that wasn't very long but took a lot of effort and running. The slight pain didn't go away but I could walk normally.

The next day at work in my high school classroom while getting up from my desk, I could not stand on my left knee and I had to spend the rest of the day in my chair and hobble to get around. The doctor reported a frayed meniscus and I wasn't able to play tennis for six weeks. Even though it was a minor injury, I didn't want to just sit around!

While I couldn't play tennis, I found I could still ride my eighteen-mile roundtrip commute on my recumbent bike. I was able to maintain a level of activity, movement, and sanity without putting my knee at risk. My knee is now fully recovered and sometimes I forget which knee was injured. I thank cycling for this recovery.

A Final Word from a Physical Therapist

Cheryl Batty is a Doctor of Physical Therapy with over 20 years' experience in orthopedic, pediatric, and neuro disciplines. Early in her career, she worked with the American Arthritis Foundation on a study comparing types of exercise considered best for managing arthritis. Although Dr. Batty is a full-time physical therapist, she finds time to teach classes at local gyms and is certified in Pilates, TRX, indoor cycling, and water aerobics. She is an active cyclist who has competed in road and mountain bike races as well as cyclo cross. After multiple knee injuries from years of ski racing, Cheryl has an intimate understanding of knee rehab and keeping knees healthy for a lifetime of function.

Two of the most common issues we treat in physical therapy are knee pain and rehab from knee surgeries. We all ask our knees to do more than almost any other joint in our bodies, since they propel us through every step we take. At some point in our lives, most of us experience knee pain. Whether this results from injury, unhealthy body weight, wear and tear, biomechanical or alignment issues, imbalances in muscle groups, sports, or even being sedentary for too long.

As we search for ways to stay active and decrease the knee pain, cycling is one of the best solutions. A no-impact activity that improves our cardio fitness, riding a bike helps stabilize the muscle groups around the knee joint and decrease the forces contributing to our pain. Bicycling also nourishes joint cartilage, which is crucial to proper knee function. There are volumes of research showing the right activity is essential to keeping our joints healthy and functioning as we age. That is probably why cycling is one of the most commonly prescribed sports to help rehab knees and balance the strength around the knee joint.

Fortunately for us, indoor cycling allows us to work out year 'round, regardless of the weather. And once a regimen becomes a habit, it's easier to translate it into our lifestyle.

It is important to begin cycle training with certified instructors. I do not recommend many cycling programs because very few follow the parameters outlined in this book. If you find a Healthy Knees Coach in your area, you are fortunate.

The *Healthy Knees Coach* and *Cycle Moles* programs lead you on a successful and injury free journey by properly fitting you to your bike and helping you through workouts designed to improve your physical and mental fitness and strength. Your trainer can also help you safely increase the challenge during the program, improve your knee and overall health, and…let you have fun doing it!

The progressions in these programs stress health for the entire body, which is crucial to moving pain free. Healthy Knees instructors devote time to working on the core as well as stretching and keeping the whole body in a fine-tuned balance. In my opinion, you can't go wrong by seeking out a Healthy Knees Coach.

History of Cycle Moles... Where did that name come from?

My home was built in the 1920s. I started my indoor training workouts in my creepy dark outside-access basement. It is one of those places where the cement floor gets wet when it rains, the narrow windows are up at the top near the low ceiling, and the spiders may just wrap you up and take you away. I guess it's kind of like a mole hole.

My husband would ask me if I was going for a "mole ride" and I'd say "yeah, I'm going for a mole ride."

Then, one day in 2008, I thought, "I don't have to do this in my dark creepy basement alone!" I'd already developed a series of progressive workouts that had improved my fitness and my knee health. I wanted to share this with others and brought Cycle Moles to Fairhaven Fitness at the Bellingham Tennis Club.

I continue to run the live training programs at the club where we fill our camps with up to 20 riders. We see an average of 10—18% increase in strength measured by watts – plus countless benefits of heart rate improvement, stronger knees and legs, and stories of feeling healthier, stronger, more energetic, and weight loss.

The Cycle Moles Training Series was born! I used the healthy knees fundamentals with the Cycle Moles groups since 2008. I formally started a "Healthy Knees Cycling" training camp in the fall of 2015 to offer a "beginners" level for those who have been inactive, haven't tried cycling, or needed guidance with their knees. It has been a huge success with all participants reporting improvement in their knees and renewed vitality.

- See more at: **http://www.cyclemoles.com/about-us**

About the Author

Robin Robertson and her husband Doug have owned and managed the Bellingham Tennis Club and Fairhaven Fitness since 2000, in Bellingham, Washington. Robin is accomplished in a variety of fitness training methods including USA Cycling Coach Level 2, Functional Aging Specialist, ACE certified personal trainer, and founder of Healthy Knees Cycling, Healthy Knees Coach, and Cycle Moles.

Robin is a life-long athlete. She ran competitively in high school and continued through college. At just 24 years old, during her senior year, she received the crushing news: if she wanted to walk at age 30, she needed to stop all impact sports because of the arthritis in her knees. Not one to take "No" for an answer, Robin turned to cycling. A new love was found!

Her first knee surgery was at the young age of 13 to correct a congenital meniscus condition and she has had a total of eight surgeries to date. Not daunted by poor knees, Robin toured the world on her bike, raced road bicycles. At ages 47 and 48, she was 2nd and 1st place Washington State "Best All Around Road Rider" Masters B Division and placed high in many other road racing events. She also raced mountain bikes and competed in the Leadville 100, among others.

She continues to train for cycling events, fitness, commutes to work, and rides her bike just for fun and to keep her knees in good health. When she's not cycling or helping others live healthy and active lives, Robin loves family time with her husband and two children, traveling, getting her hands dirty in her garden, and sewing (Halloween costumes are her favorite).

You can find out more about Robin, Healthy Knees Cycling, Cycle Moles, and the Bellingham Tennis Club and Fairhaven Fitness at the following:

www.HealthyKneesBook.com
www.CycleMoles.com
www.BellinghamTennis.com
www.FairhavenFitness.us

APPENDIX:
KNOW YOUR KNEES
(A Short Anatomy Lesson)

Understanding Knees and a Few Fun Facts

In the human body, a joint is where two or more bones come together. We humans have about 230 of them! They have different ranges of movement including no mobility, limited movement, and full range of movement. Joint action is classified by type such as ball and socket, hip and saddle joints, or a hinge (like the knee). Joints can also be classified by structure, function, biomechanical properties and more – it really gets very technical.

Your knee is the largest and most complex of the joints that are made for free movement. It primarily acts like a hinge and when flexed is capable of some rotation and lateral movement. There are four directional terms you should know: medial is toward your mid-line or the center of your body; lateral is away from the mid line or to sides of your body; anterior is toward the front of your body; posterior is toward the backside of your body.

Regardless of the classification, joints would not function very well if they were just bone meeting bone. There would be too much friction! Similar to a ball bearing sealed with oil, human joints that move have a joint capsule containing either cartilage or synovial fluid – or both – between the bones to allow for ease of movement. Cartilage is a smooth, tough connective tissue pad to absorb impact between bones; synovial fluid is a yolk-like viscous substance that lubricates the joint.

Bones of the Knee and Leg

Let's start with your leg bones. Three bones meet to form your knee: femur (thigh bone), tibia (the shin bone), and patella (kneecap). Starting at the top of your leg, the hip end of your femur has two knobs. One knob is the "ball" for the ball and socket of your hip joint. The other is a bony protuberance called the Greater Trochanter where your gluteal muscles (and others) are attached to help rotate your thigh. Your femur ends at your knee with two knobs (called condyles) of the knee joint.

These two knee condyles of the femur rest on the top of your tibia (your biggest of two lower leg bones) on the tibial plateau. The fibula (the smaller of two lower leg bones) is nestled to the lateral side of your tibia. It sits underneath the tibial plateau. At the foot end of your shin, your tibia and fibula connect into the bones of your foot and your ankle bone is the end of your fibula.

Fun fact: your femur is the longest bone in your body

Your kneecap is called the patella. It stays in its place because it is imbedded in the large quadriceps femoral tendon and anchored to the tibia with the patellar ligament (commonly called the patellar tendon).

Fun fact: not all people have a patella. The patella is a "sesamoid" bone and only grows out of irritation, but most people have them.

Cartilage Cushions

Your knee has two types of cartilage: articular cartilage and fibrocartilage.

The real cushions of the knee are the two C-shaped menisci cartilage which sit on the tibial plateau between the femur and tibia. The menisci act as a shock absorber and are made of dense, fibrocartilage that is sort of like memory foam: it continually changes shape to adapt to the movement of the knee, but returns to its original shape. The menisci also help to stabilize the knee in medial and lateral movements (side to side).

Articular cartilage is like a shrink-wrap padded protection for bones. The knee side of your patella has the thickest articular cartilage in your whole body. This is because the kneecap takes more pressure per unit of area than any other part of the body. The ends of your bones are shrink-wrapped with articular cartilage for added protection.

Fun fact: Lunges and squats can produce pressure of up to six times your bodyweight onto your kneecap[23]

Another Fun Fact: Meniscus comes from the Greek word for "crescent." Each meniscus cartilage is a wedge-shaped crescent with the thick edges toward the outsides of your knee.

Ligaments and Tendons: the "Ropes" Holding it Together

Ligaments attach bone to bone and tendons attach muscle to bone.

The most famous of your knee ligaments are the cruciate ligaments. Inside the knee joint are the two ligaments, crossing each other like an "X," connecting the femur to the tibia: the Anterior Cruciate Ligament (ACL) is toward the front of the knee and the Posterior Cruciate Ligament (PCL) is behind it. Tears to the ACL are often seen in injuries from soccer and skiing. Besides keeping your bones connected and in place, your ACL is responsible for preventing your knee from hyperextension; the PCL's job is to prevent hyperflexion.

Fun fact: "cruciate" means "cross."

The other ligaments of your knee include the collateral ligaments on the sides. These provide stability and brace your knee against unusual movement. The lateral (fibular) collateral ligament stabilizes the outside and the medial (tibial) collateral ligament (MCL) reinforces the inside

---

[23] King. W Dr., (2015), *Chondromalacia Patella Pain in the Front Part of the Knee.* Sutter Health Palo Alto Medical Foundation. Retrieved 9/21/15 from **http://www.pamf.org/sports/king/condromaliciapatella.html**

of your knee. The MCL is also connected to your medial meniscus. An injury to this ligament usually affects the medial meniscus as well.

Two Joints in One

The knee joint is constructed of two compartmentalized joints. The Tibiofemoral joint is what we often think of as the knee. It includes the area where the thigh bone (femur) meets the shin bone (tibia). The Patellofemoral joint is where the kneecap (patella) meets the femur.

Inside the tibiofemoral joint is the joint capsule. The joint capsule is lined with the synovial membrane which produces the synovial joint fluid that lubricates the knee, your menisci, and cruciate ligaments.